Photo Diagnosis

for Passing the
USMLE
Steps 1, 2 & 3

Vol. II

Second Edition

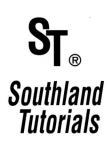

**Southland
Tutorials**

CONTRIBUTORS

Stanley Gold, M.D.
Jeffrey Birnbaum, M.D.
Michael Wagner,, M D.
Gloria Thompson, M.D.
Melvin Jackson, M.D.
Carol Henneman, M.D.
Lorraine Walker, M.D.
Michael Donahue, M.D.
Daniel Levine, M.D.
Corrine Wilson, M.D.

CONTENTS

INTRODUCTION

Photodiagnosis for Passing the USMLE Steps 1,2 & 3, Vol II, is designed to help medical students and physicians preparing for the USMLE. It is a study aid to test and improve your diagnostic skills in the broad range of basic and clinical science cases in the USMLE.

This is the first photodiagnosis prepared specifically for those preparing for the USMLE. The variety of cases which appear in this homestudy course represent problems common in these examinations. Although the spectrum of cases is extensive, it is not exhaustive but will fill an important gap for the reader.

A carefully selected photograph or a diagram is easier to assimilate than written text, and is easier to recall under examination conditions. This has been written as a simple revision text, and includes basic and clinical science photographs, x-rays, EKGs, and gross pathology.

The questions have been designed to be brief and to the point, while the answers are extensive to include the differential diagnoses. When you look at a photograph for the first time, always reconsider the first thing that comes to your mind and test it against logical deduction: if it appears wrong do not discard it totally, often the first thought is right!

It is hoped that this photodiagnosis will prove of particular value to the candidates taking the USMLE Steps 1,2 & 3. These pictorial tests when used in conjunction with our other homestudy courses will improve your scores in these examinations.

SOUTHLAND TUTORIALS

Second Edition

PHOTO DIAGNOSIS

QUESTIONS

Vol. 2

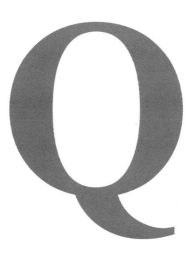

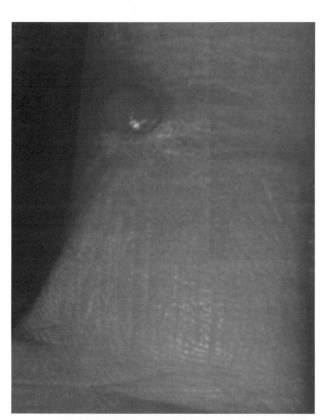

1. For several months, a 12-year-old boy has had a lesion on the fourth digit of his left hand that at first resembled a common wart. Although the lesion is not painful or pruritic, it became irritated and began to bleed two weeks after his mother began to apply an over-the-counter wart medication. On examination, you find a shiny red, friable tumor on the palmar aspect of the finger.

What is your diagnosis?

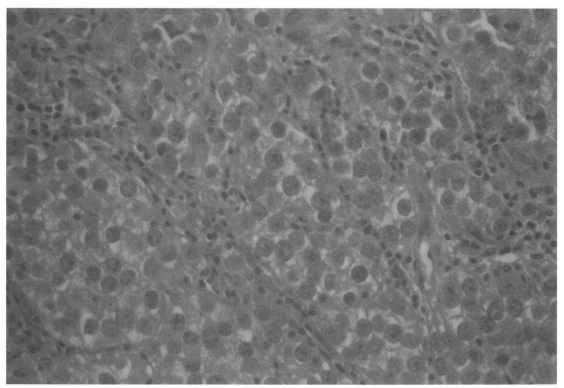

2. A 40-year-old man presented with painless, progressive unilateral testicular enlargement. A homogeneous, soft, pale tan-gray mass, 5 cm in diameter and nearly replacing the testes, was excised.

What is your diagnosis?

A. Teratocarcinoma   C. Malignant lymphoma
B. Seminoma   D. Interstitial cell tumor

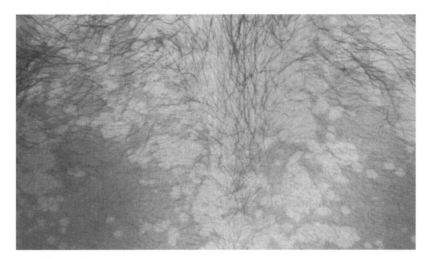

3. A 20-year-old man is worried about some asymtomatic pale spots that appeared over his chest, back, shoulders, and arms several months ago. He's been out in the sun a lot since then, and the contrast between the tanned normal skin and the untanned patches has become striking and embarrassing. Examination reveals fine, hypopigmented macules and confluent patches.

What is your diagnosis?

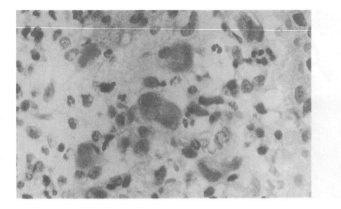 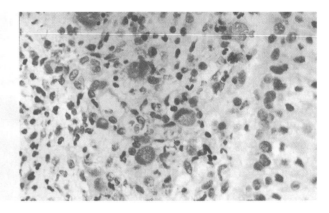

4. A 30-year-old HIV-infected homosexual man presented with a three week history of odynophagia and dysphagia to solids and liquids. Esophagogastroduodenoscopy showed multiple, small, 0.5-cm ulcers in the lower two-thirds of the esophagus. His stomach and duodenum were normal. Biopsy of the ulcers was performed.

What is your diagnosis?

A. Herpesvirus infection   C. Cytomegalovirus infection
B. *Candida* esophagitis   D. Reflux esophagitis

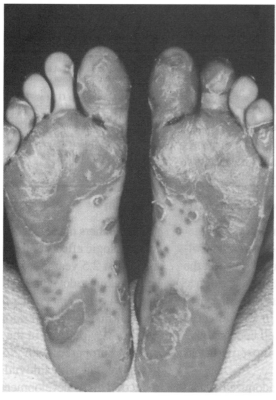 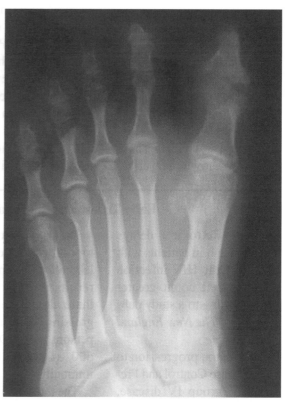

5. A 23-year-old heterosexual man presented to the emergency department with epigastric and left-sided chest pain. Subsequent cardiac evaluation was noncontributory. There was a five- to six-year history of swollen feet and recurrent bouts of urethritis. Physical exam revealed the plantar rash pictured above, as well as a similar rash on the penis and scrotum, erythematous papules of the tongue, and swollen, erythematous toes. X-ray of the left foot is also shown.

What is your diagnosis?

A. Arthritis-dermatitis syndrome   C. Gout   E. Reiter's syndrome
B. Psoriatic arthritis   D. Kawasaki disease

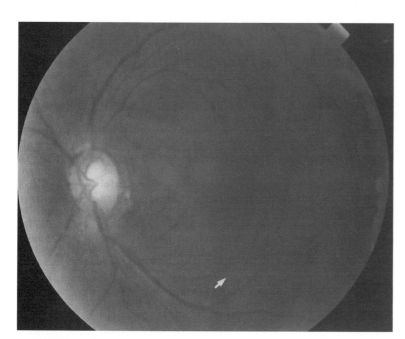

6. A 66-year-old female psychiatric patient presented with a complaint of gradually decreasing visual acuity, which was more prominent in the evening.

What is your diagnosis?

A. Cytomegalovirus retinitis
B. Retinitis pigmentosa, early-onset
C. Early thioridazine toxicity
D. Diabetic retinopathy

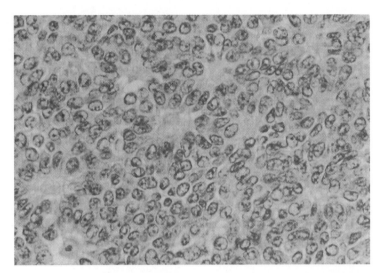

7. A 64-year-old woman was admitted with complaints of postmenopausal bleeding and lower abdominal pain. Pelvic examination revealed an enlarged uterus (the size of a 14-week pregnancy). Abdominal ultrasound showed a right-sided adnexal mass free of the uterus. Endometrial curettage showed cystic hyperplasia.

What is your diagnosis?

A. Adenocarcinoma of the ovary   C. Carcinoid tumor   E. Theca cell tumor
B. Endometrial stromal sarcoma   D. Granulosa cell tumor

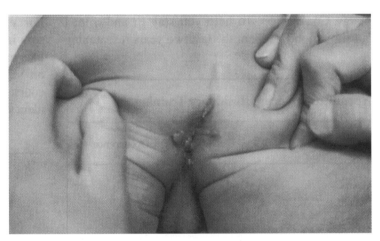

8. A six-month-old boy was noted to have a warty growth in the perianal area.

What is your diagnosis?

A. Molluscum contagiosum
B. Condylomata acuminata
C. Genital herpes
D. Condylomata lata of secondary syphilis

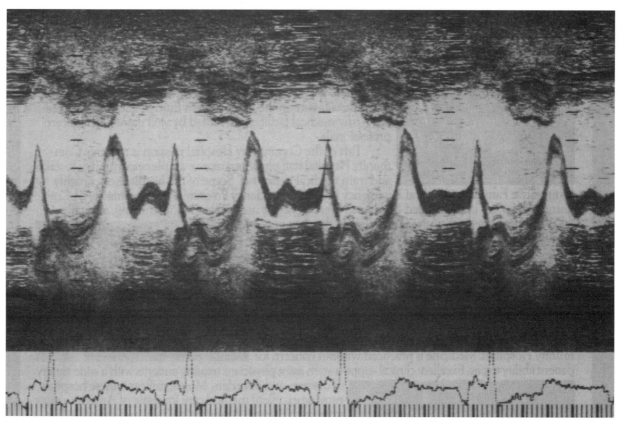

9. A 51-year-old man presented with palpitations. He had been informed of a heart murmur in the past, but he had no evaluation. After an initial evaluation, an echocardiogram was obtained.

What is your diagnosis?

A. Mitral valve prolapse
B. Bacterial endocarditis
C. Normal study
D. Mitral stenosis

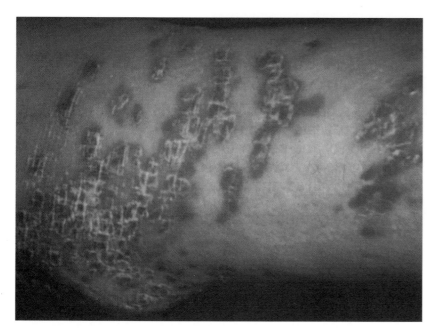

10. A 62-year-old male from Southern Europe has had this eruption for about 12 years. He has no pruritus and is asymptomatic.

What is your diagnosis?

A. Lichen planus
B. Kaposi's sarcoma
C. Psoriasis
D. Chronic fungus infection

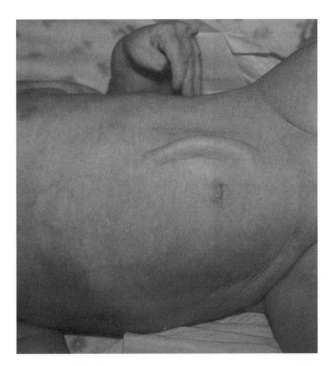

11. A six-month-old boy is brought to the office because he has had watery diarrhea and has been vomiting and not eating well for the past five days. On examination, the irritable infant has poor skin turgor and noticeably decreased peripheral perfusion. His saliva is sticky and mucous membranes dry, and both his fontanelle and his eyeballs are sunken. The infant's blood pressure is 85/35 mm Hg, respiratory rate 60, and heart rate 120 beats a minute. His chest is clear to auscultation, and the rest of the physical examination is unremarkable. Laboratory studies show a serum sodium of 128 mmol/L, potassium 4.6 mmol/L, chloride 95 mmol/L, and total carbon dioxide 15 mmol/L.

What is your diagnosis?

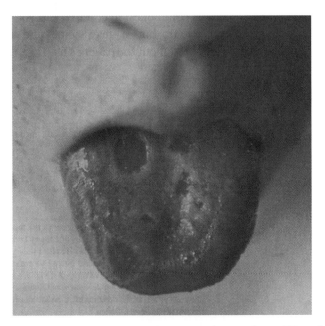

12. The tongue of a 10-year-old girl has ridges and patches over its surface. The girl has no lingual pain or other symptoms, but the unsightly problem has recurred several times in the past few years. Her physical examination is otherwise unremarkable.

What is your diagnosis?

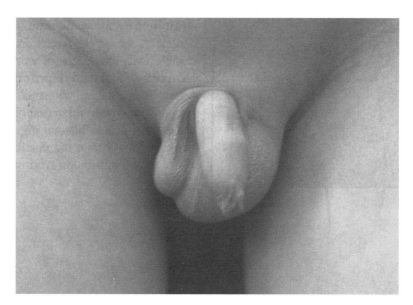

13. A six-year-old boy comes into the office with a mass in the left side of the scrotum. The mass, which appeared eight months ago, gets bigger when he cries, strains, or coughs but recedes when he lies down. It disappears entirely when compressed. The boy has no associated abdominal pain, vomiting, or diarrhea.

What is your diagnosis?

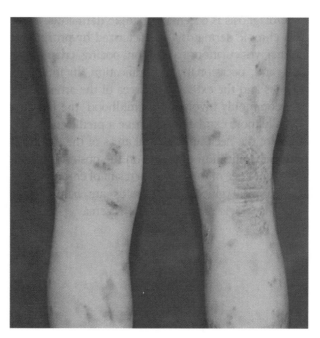

14. A six-year-old boy has had a generalized, intermittent, and itchy rash for 18 months. Initially, the lesions were erythematous, weeping, and oozing. More recently, the lesions became thickened, dry, and scaly. Physical examination shows scaly and pigmented lesions on the trunk and extremities. The lesions are more prominent on the flexural aspects of the arms and legs.

What is your diagnosis?

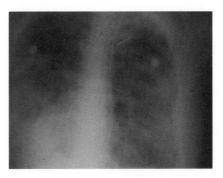

15. A 63-year-old man presented with fever, shortness of breath, and a relentless cough. Despite intensive antibiotic and general supportive therapy, he died 10 days after the onset of symtoms.
The x-ray findings are most consistent with the diagnosis of:

A. Pneumonia
B. Tuberculosis
C. Pulmonary fibrosis
D. Lung cancer

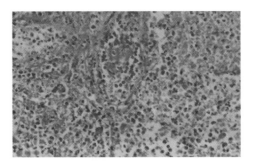

16. These histologic features are most compatible with the diagnosis of:

A. Bacterial pneumonia
B. Viral pneumonia
C. Pneumocystis carinii pneumonitis
D. Shock lung

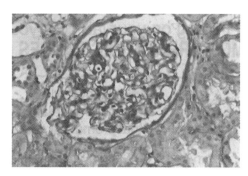

17. This photograph shows the light microscopic appearance of a typical glomerulus from the kidney biopsy of a patient who presented with microhematuria and proteinuria. All the other glomeruli looked like the one here. On the basis of these light microscopic findings, the most likely diagnosis is:

A. Poststreptococcal glomerulonephritis
B. Membranoproliferative glomerulonephritis
C. Crecentic glomerulonephritis
D. Mesangial nephropathy (Berger's disease)

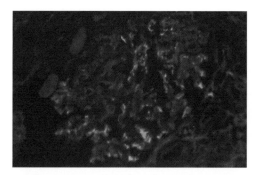

18.   The diagnosis of mesangial nephropathy (Berger's disease) was confirmed by immunofluorescence microscopy. The deposits, seen as brightly fluorescent streaks and granules in the mesangial areas of this glomerulus, contain:

A. IgA
B. Fibrin
C. C1q component of complement
D. IgE

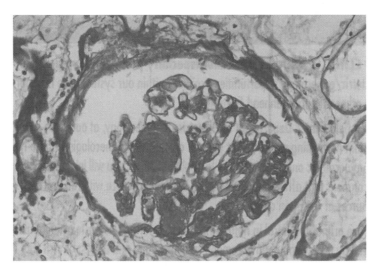

19. A 48-year-old obese woman was admitted to the hospital in a hypotensive state, with sepsis, proteinuria, and a high blood urea nitrogen level. She had a history of congestive heart failure, chronic renal failure, and noninsulin-dependent diabetes mellitus. She died after ten days in the hospital.

What is your diagnosis?

A. Chronic pyelonephritis   C. Amyloid nephropathy
B. Arteriolonephrosclerosis   D. Nodular glomerulosclerosis

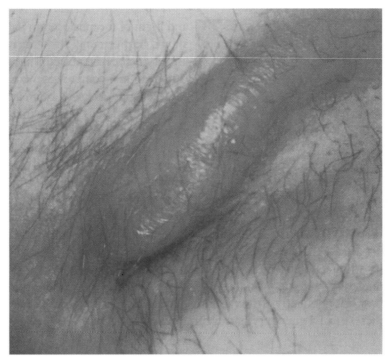

20. A 41-year-old man complains of recurrent painful "boils" he's had on and off in both armpits for several years. Otherwise in good health, he takes no medications. No one in his family has had boils, but his mother and grandmother have controlled diabetes. He uses roll-on deodorants when the pain is not severe. Examination reveals large, tender, erythematous, fluctuant abscess in both axillae, especially on the right.

What is your diagnosis?

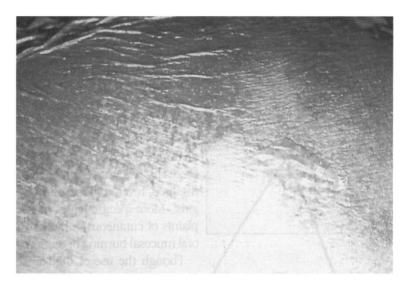

21. A 55-year-old woman is brought to the emergency department for evaluation of a sudden rash. One week ago, she was given a sulfa drug for dysuria. Her genitourinary symptoms resolved, but a widespread morbilliform eruption developed, and last night she complained of severe skin and mouth pain along with blisters over her trunk. On examination, she is febrile and has diffuse skin tenderness. Numerous erythematous macules and patches of various sizes and scattered flaccid and partially ruptured bullae are found over much of her body, though her face and scalp have been relatively spared. With lateral pressure on the erythematous skin, the epidermis separates from the underlying dermis.

What is your diagnosis?

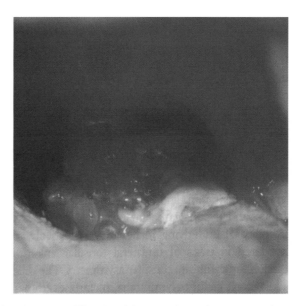

22. A 61-year-old man is brought to your office by his daughter for evaluation of a chronic left-sided sore throat accompanied by a sensation of a lump in the throat; occasionally, he has an associated earache as well. His daughter is particularly worried because her father has been treated unsuccessfully with antibiotics for more than six months. On examination, you find a large exophytic mass on the left tonsil and a palpable neck mass on the same side.

What is your diagnosis?

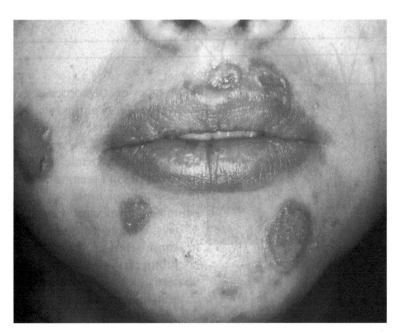

23. A 12-year-old boy has a "rash" that began as a single pustule over his right cheek two weeks ago and has spread to his chin and mouth. The erosions are somewhat pruritic, slightly tender to the touch, and covered with a honey-colored crust. The boy has a few tender anterior cervical nodes.

What is your diagnosis?

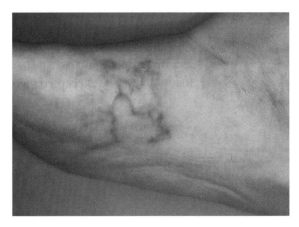

24. A 21-year-old woman who recently returned from a trip to Mexico complains of a pruritic eruption on her foot that developed a few days after she arrived there. She says she spent most of her time at the beach. The eruption has spread, is intensely itchy, and consists of a thin, serpiginous, somewhat elevated burrow over the medial and plantar aspects of the anterior portion of her right foot. Several areas have become crusted and excoriated. She is otherwise in good health.

What is your diagnosis?

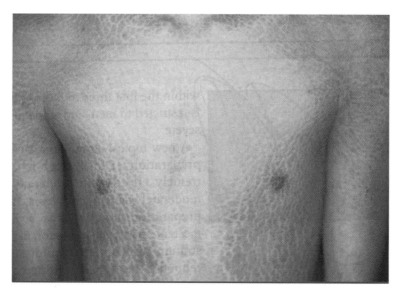

25. An 18-year-old man has had a dry, scaly, generalized eruption since the age of six months. It consists of discrete, shiny scales with a "pasted-on" look, most prominent over his trunk and lower legs. The edges of the scales are slightly raised. The eruption has spared his face, neck, and antecubital and popliteal fossae. There is slight accentuation of the palmar and plantar skin markings. Various creams and ointments have been of little help. His father and brother have a similar condition, and in all three the dryness and scaling get worse in the colder months.

What is your diagnosis?

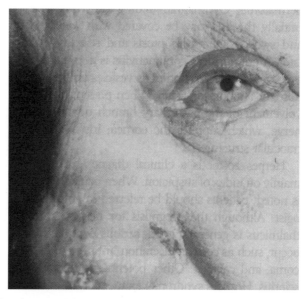

26. A 73-year-old man, otherwise in good health, comes to the office with a painful rash affecting his left lower eyelid, left cheek, and the tip of his nose. Three days earlier he noticed mild redness of the eye, blurred vision, lid swelling, and discomfort with bright lights. Examination of the eye discloses ptosis and conjunctivitis.

What is your diagnosis?

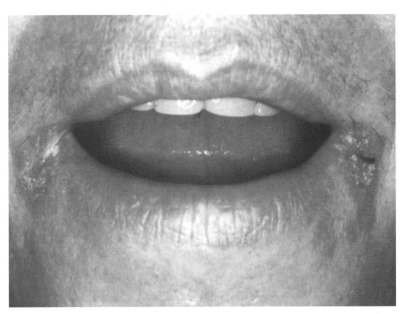

27. A 55-year-old woman has had painful cracks in the corners of her mouth intermittently for the past several months. No proprietary medications have helped. She wears dentures, which she says "have to be replaced." A triangular area of erythema and edema with fissuring is visible at each mouth angle.

What is your diagnosis?

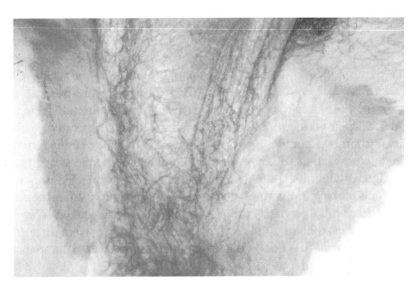

28. A 31-year-old man complains of an itchy rash in his groin that has worsened in the past few weeks. A variety of over-the-counter antipruritic medications have failed to relieve him. Examination reveals a fairly well demarcated, hyperpigmented eruption with somewhat raised and erythematous borders. The patient also has a marked ringworm infection of his feet.

What is your diagnosis?

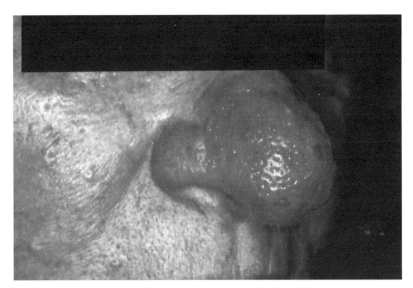

29. A 57-year-old man complains that his nose, which has been red and greasy for the past two years, has become increasingly large. He is embarrassed by his appearance, and since he does not consume alcoholic beverages, he is worried that his condition may herald a malignancy. Greasy masses of firm, thick, lobulated, reddish purple tissue cover the nose.

What is your diagnosis?

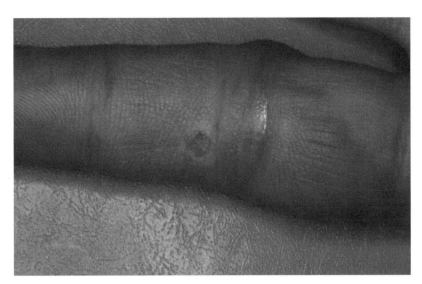

30. A 54-year-old Asian cook has a reddish purple edematous eruption with a sharply defined scalloped advancing border that developed after he pricked his right middle finger on a shrimp shell while at work. He is otherwise in good health, but the lesion is painful and has begun to interfere with his work.

 What is your diagnosis?

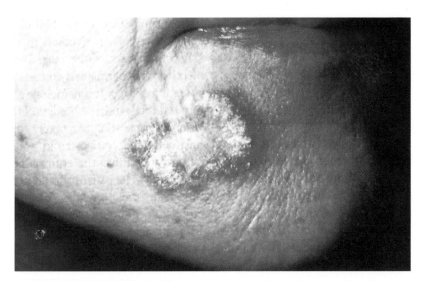

31. A 47-year-old woman has a nonpruritic rash over the left side of her chin. The rash has been spreading in the past few months. She is apparently in good health and takes no medications.

What is your diagnosis?

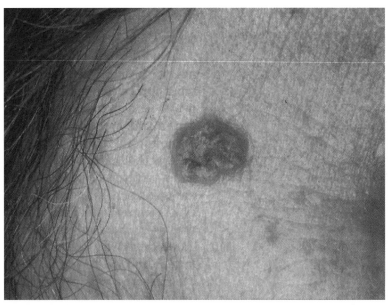

32. A 57-year-old woman has a sore on the right side of her face. It has not healed, and when traumatized by excessive hair brushing, it occasionally bleeds. She has no subjective symptoms, but the sore has begun to grow and she is worried that it might be a cancer. On examination, you see a round, nontender, waxy-looking 1-cm lesion with a somewhat irregular, heaped-up, pearly border. Tiny flecks of pigment are spattered throughout the lesion.

What is your diagnosis?

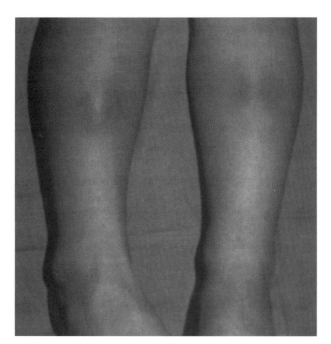

33. A 24-year-old woman complains of fever and a tender eruption on her legs. The illness began that morning, preceded by stiffness in her joints; her knees have been aching all day. Two weeks ago she had a sore throat that resolved without treatment. She has taken no aspirin, antibiotics, or oral contraceptives. Her temperature is 102.4 °F, and she appears acutely ill. Her knees are slightly swollen and erythematous; patches of extremely tender erythematous nodules are seen on the front of both legs.

What is your diagnosis?

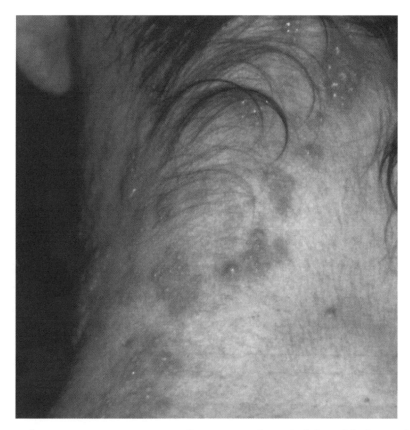

34. A 30-year-old man seeks emergency treatment for a severely painful and itchy rash that appeared over the back of his neck and scalp four or five days ago. He has not been bitten or stung by any insects, takes no medication, doesn't have any household pets, and is otherwise in good health. Except for a unilateral vesicular, erythematous eruption beginning at the right nuchal scalp and extending down to the right scapular area, the examination is within normal limits.

What is your diagnosis?

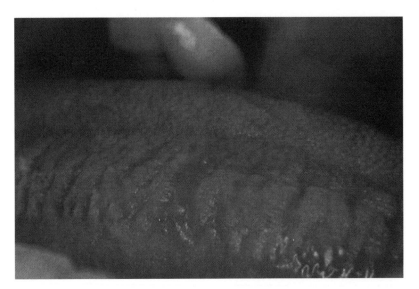

35. A 26-year-old man comes to your office because his tongue has been white and fuzzy along the sides for the past three months. It has not produced any symptoms, and although he has been losing weight recently, has felt somewhat fatigued, and has occasional night sweats, he claims to be in good health. An enzyme-linked immunosorbent assay for HIV is positive.

What is your diagnosis?

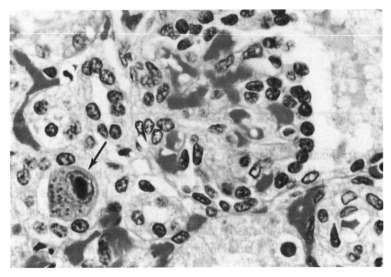

36. An infant boy was born to a mother who was an intravenous drug-abuser. The pregnancy and delivery were uneventful. The baby died after one week in the hospital.

What is your diagnosis?

A. Herpes infection   C. Rubella
B. Cytomegalovirus infection   D. Measles

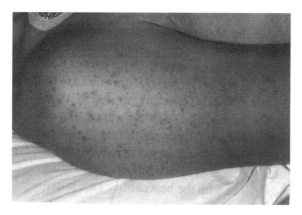

37. A 24-year-old man was admitted to the hospital for *Hymenoptera* venom desensitization. The patient had been on oral corticosteroids for one week because of a recent bee sting and suffered a severe reaction. While being desensitized, he had an anaphylactic reaction and required aggressive treatment that included high doses of systemic corticosteroids. A few days later, a diffuse, asymptomatic pustular rash appeared on his trunk and upper arms.

What is your diagnosis?

A. Acne vulgaris   C. Steroid-induced acne   E. Disseminated herpes zoster

B. Miliaria (prickly heat)   D. Folliculitis

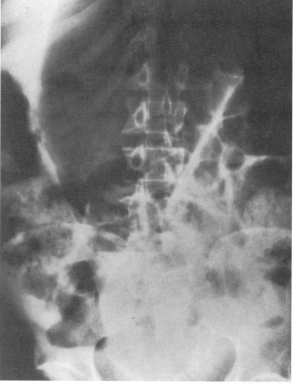

38. A 67-year-old man has abdominal pain and distention. What is your interpretation of the supine (left) and upright (right) films of his abdomen?

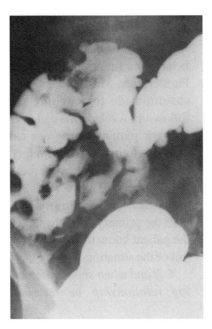

39. A 46-year-old woman was admitted to the hospital because of generalized abdominal pain, nausea, substernal pain, and vomiting. Six months previously, she had been operated on for intestinal obstruction and had lost 14 kg of body weight during the past three months. Her arterial blood pressure was 120/80 mmHg. The abdomen was soft, and no palpable mass was detected. The laboratory tests were within normal limits, except for the hematocrit (36%). The ultrasound examination was negative.

What is your diagnosis?

A. Postsurgical adhesions of the colon
B. Diffuse gastric carcinoma infiltrating the colon
C. Annular carcinoma of the colon
D. Colonic lymphoma
E. Colonic tuberculosis

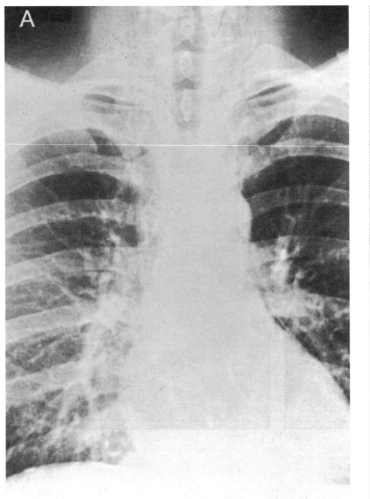
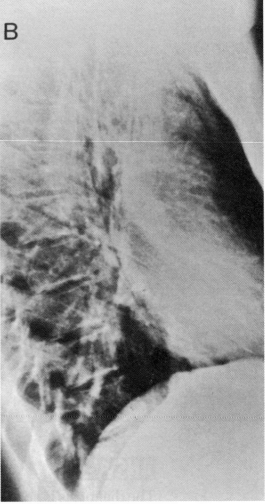

40. A 20-year-old man had a sudden onset of chest pain while lifting weights and was taken to an emergency department for evaluation. What is your interpretation of his chest films?

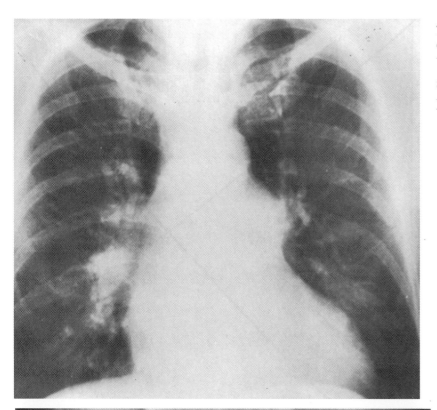

41. A 65-year-old man with a history of coronary insufficiency has had shortness of breath and a cough for three days. His lungs seem unremarkable on auscultation. What is your interpretation of his chest film?

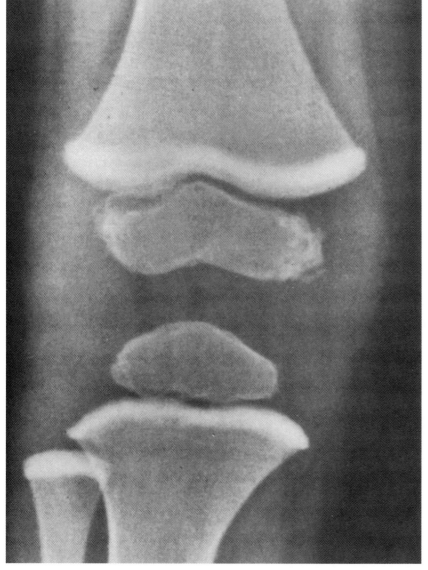

42. A two-year-old, poorly nourished girl has a swollen right knee after a fall. The knee is slightly ecchymotic anteriorly. What is your interpretation of the frontal film of her knee?

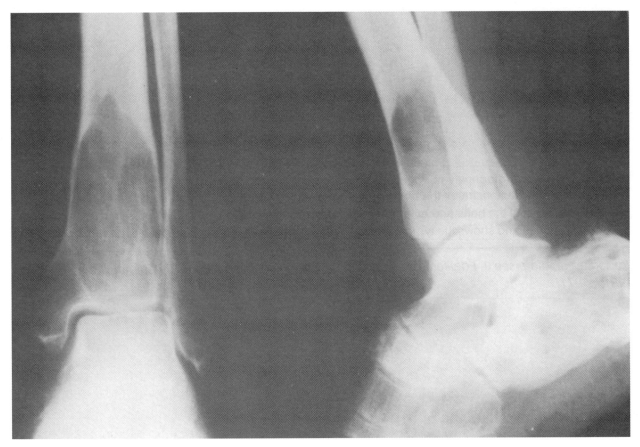

43. A 70-year-old man complains of pain of six months duration in his left ankle. Physical examination is unremarkable. What is your interpretation of the frontal (left) and lateral (right) views of his ankle?

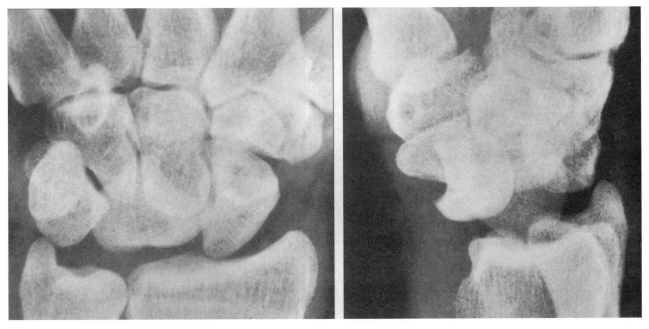

44. A 38-year-old man fell on his outstretched hand. What is your interpretation of the frontal and lateral views of his left wrist?

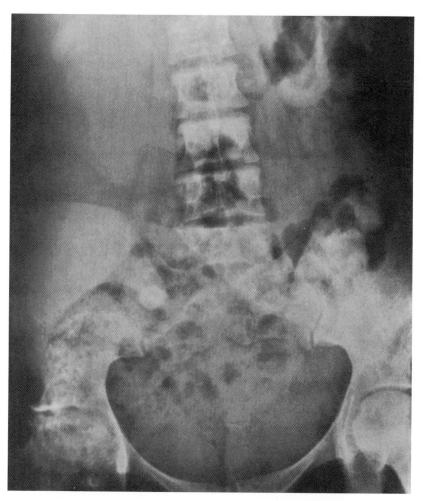

45. A 35-year-old black woman has had abdominal pain for the past six hours. The abdomen is diffusely tender to palpation. What is your interpretation of the scout film of her abdomen?

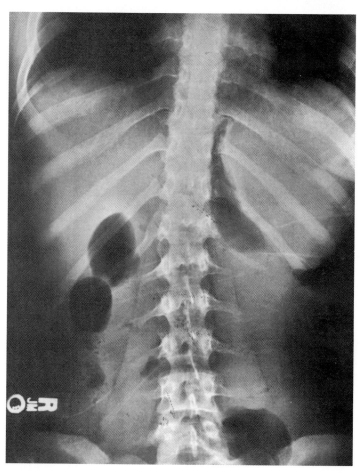

46. A 27-year-old woman with a history of drug abuse complains of abdominal pain. No further history is immediately available. Moderate epigastric tenderness with minimal guarding is found on abdominal examination. What is your interpretation of the scout film of her abdomen?

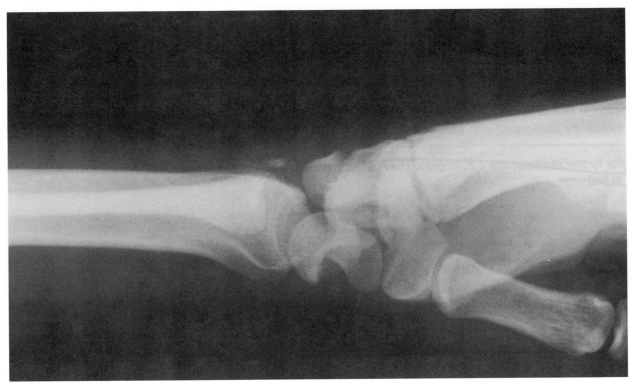

47. A 25-year-old man fell on his outstreched hand. His wrist is painful and swollen. What is your interpretation of the wrist film?

48. A 20-year-old man has had foot pain for three months. Examination reveals tenderness over the head of his second metatarsal. What is your interpretation of the x-ray?

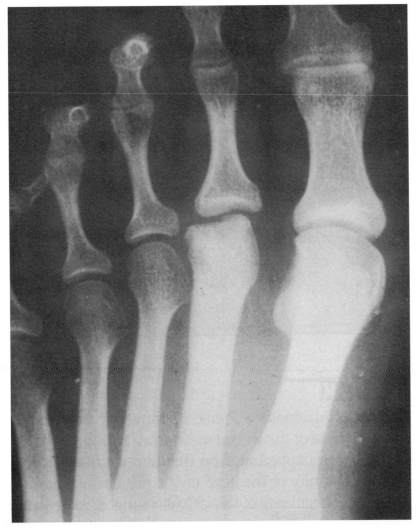

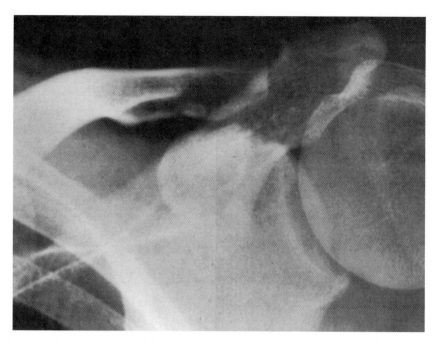

49. After being injured in an auto accident, a 30-year-old man has pain and limitation of movement in his shoulder. What is your interpretation of the frontal film of his shoulder?

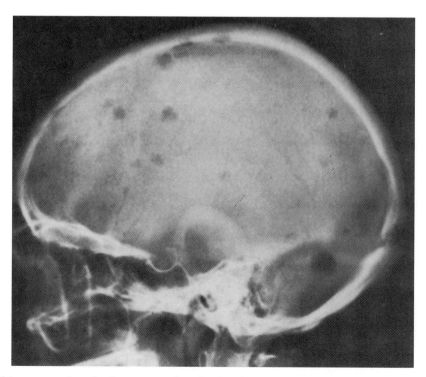

50. A 60-year-old woman has had a severe headache for a week. What is your interpretation of the lateral skull projection?

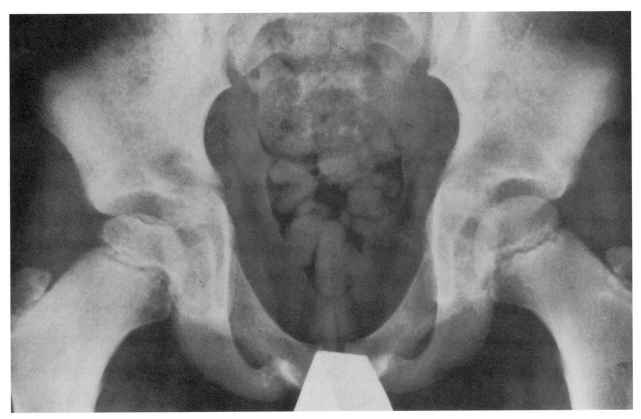

51. For several months, a 10-year-old boy has been complaining of pain in his right hip. What is your interpretation of the frontal film of his pelvis?

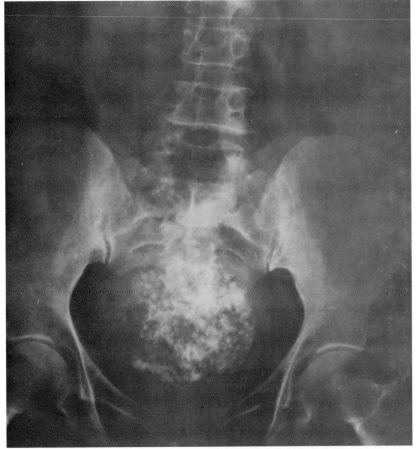

52. A 60-year-old woman is examined and found to have a pelvic mass. What is your interpretation of her abdominal scout film?

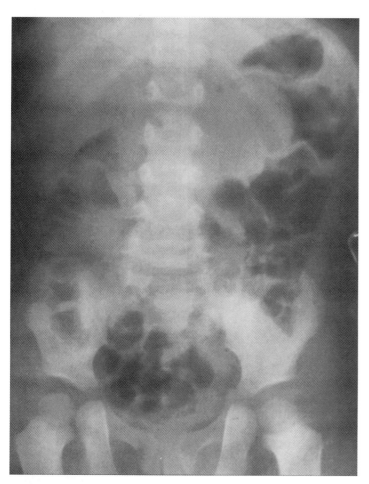

53. A two-year-old girl complains of abdominal pain. According to her parents, the pain has been intermittent for about four hours. Her abdomen is tender to palpation and bowel sounds are hyperactive. What is your interpretation of the scout film of her abdomen?

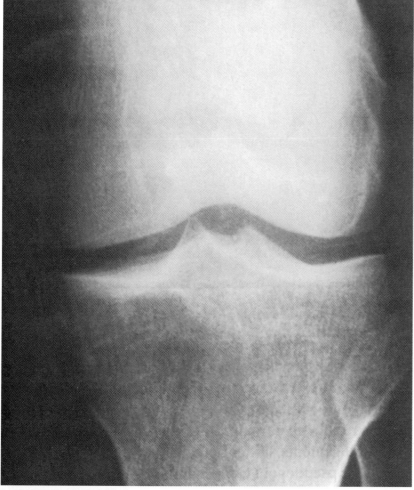

54. A 54-year-old man has had marked inflammation and pain in his knee for several days. What is your interpretation of the knee film?

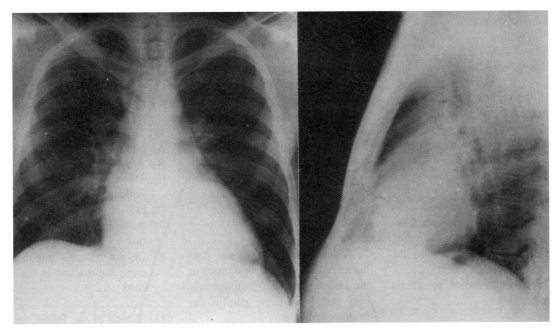

55. This chest roentgenogram shows an AP view on the left and a left lateral view.

What is your diagnosis?

A. Left ventricular hypertrophy and congestive heart failure
B. Calcification of the mitral valve
C. Calcification of a left ventricular aneurysm or left ventricular wall
D. Dissecting aneurysm
E. Calcified pericardium with possible constriction

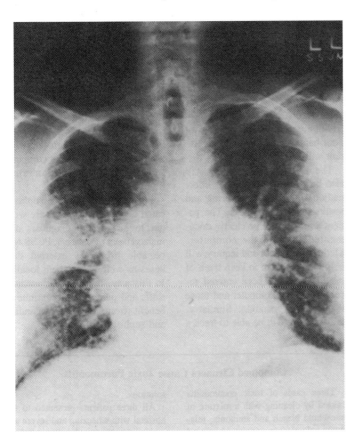

56. This 46-year-old malnourished man was admitted in a semicomatose condition with a high fever, profuse night sweats, and headaches. Meningeal signs were absent. Total white cell count was 3,800/µL with bandemia.

What is your diagnosis?

A. Chickenpox pneumonia
B. Hemosiderosis
C. Miliary tuberculosis
D. Loeffler's syndrome
E. Multiple secondaries

Right Ventricle

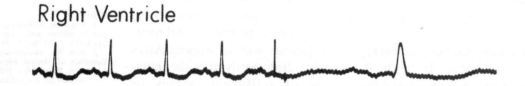

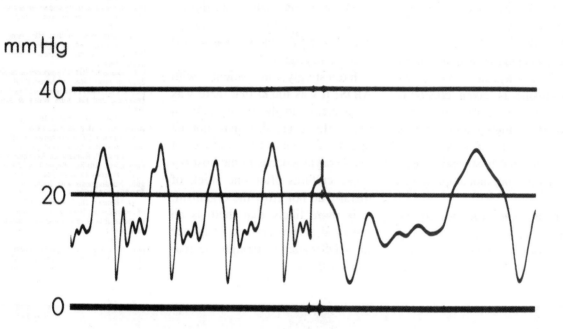

57. In this pressure tracing from the right ventricle, the electrocardiogram is on the top and the pressure tracing appears on the bottom. The last portion of the record was run at high speed.

What is your diagnosis?

A. Pulmonic stenosis   C. Pulmonary embolism   E. Mitral stenosis
B. Tricuspid stenosis   D. Constrictive pericarditis

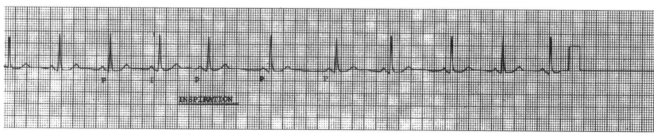

58. The irregularity in the cardiac rhythm seen in an otherwise healthy, 35-year-old active male is due to one of the following:

What is your diagnosis?

A. Wenckebach block   C. Atrial fibrillation
B. Sinus arrhythmia   D. Atrial flutter

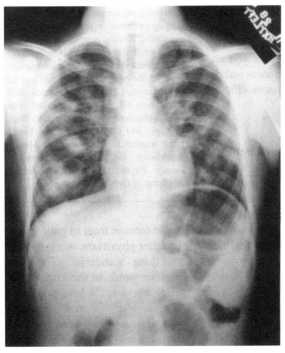
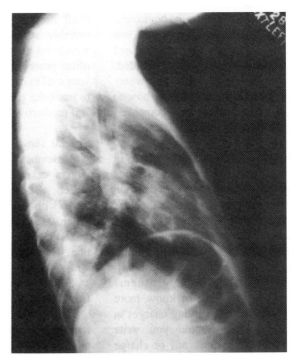

59. A seven-year-old male presented with chest pain.

What is your diagnosis?

A. Wegener's granulomatosis
B. Streptococcal pnuemonia with abscess formation
C. Histiocytosis X
D. Metastases

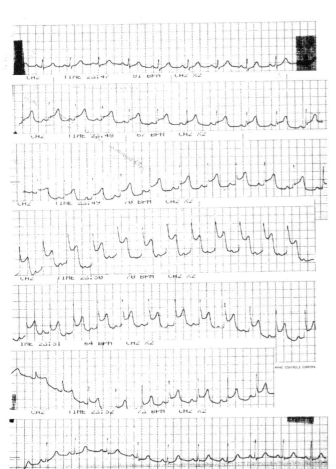

60. A 51-year-old woman presented with nocturnal chest pain. A graded exercise test revealed no evidence of ischemia. A Holter monitor recording was performed, and representative tracings are shown below.

What is your diagnosis?

A. Prinzmetal's angina
B. Acute myocardial infarction
C. Paroxysmal ventricular tachycardia
D. Pericarditis

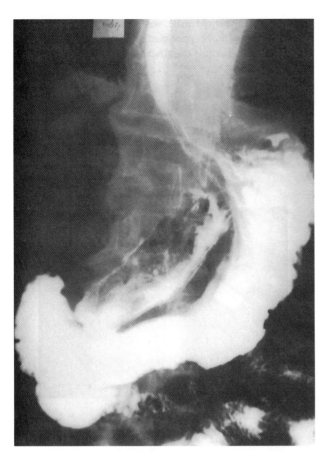

61. An 82-year-old man suffered from melena for four days before being admitted to the hospital. He had experienced another episode of melena the previous summer. On examination we found edema, cardiac failure, and a positive fecal blood test. The hematocrit was 24%, and the white cell count was 22,000, with 90% neutrophils and 10% lymphocytes. Seven days later he underwent an exploratory laparotomy. Barium meal x-ray is shown.

What is your diagnosis?

A. Gastric diverticula
B. Lymphoma
C. Perforation of gastric ulcer
D. Bezoar of the stomach

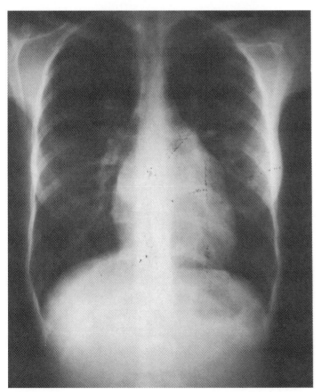

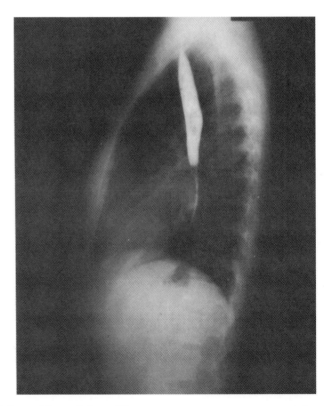

62. This 25-year-old woman complained of difficult, labored breathing. Chest roentgenograms were taken.

What is your diagnosis?

A. Atrial septal defect   C. Aortic insufficiency   E. Cardiomyopathy
B. Mitral stenosis   D. Ventricular septal defect

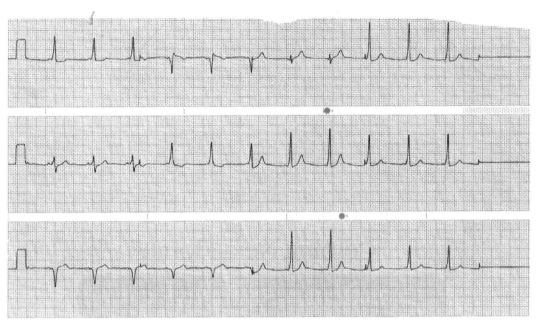

63. Which of the following syndromes is most commonly associated with this electrocardiogram?

A. Barlow's syndrome
B. Wolff-Parkinson-White syndrome

C. Tietze's syndrome
D. Lown-Ganong-Levine syndrome

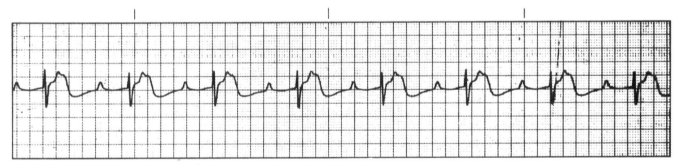

64. This rhythm strip was obtained on the second day of an I.C.U. hospitalization of a 43-year-old man with an acute anterior myocardial infarction. Which of the following is the correct rhythm?

A. First-degree heart block
B. Second-degree heart block (Mobitz Type I) Wenckebach

C. Second-degree heart block (Mobitz Type II)
D. Complete heart block

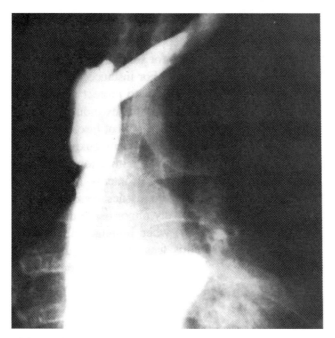 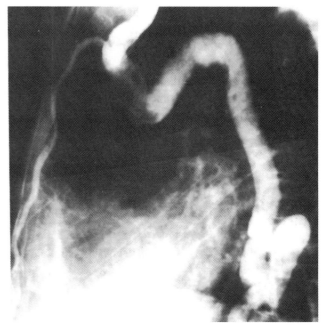

65. This man was in his 40s and had biopsy-proven and cultured actinomycosis of his mediastinum.

What is your diagnosis?

A. Coarctation of the aorta   D. Obstruction of superior vena cava with collateral circulation
B. Left superior vena cava   E. Patent vein bypass
C. Carotid artery aneurysm

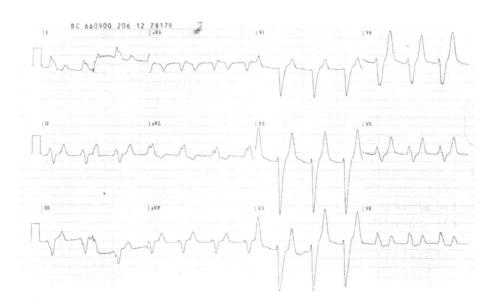

66. This abnormal ECG seen in a 70-year-old man is due to which of the following?

A. Acute myocardial infarction
B. Hyperkalemia
C. Acute pericarditis
D. Normal variant

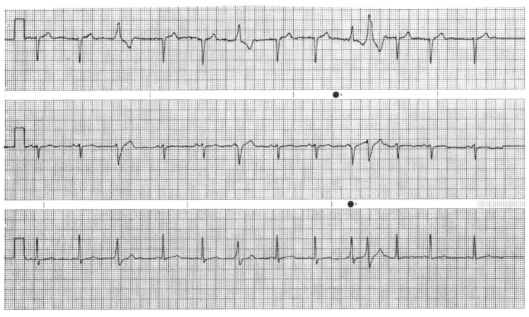

67. Which of the following cardiovascular pharmacotherapeutic agents is the most likely etiologic agent of the dysrhythmia shown on the rhythm strip?

A. Quinidine   C. Propanolol
B. Digoxin   D. Xylocaine

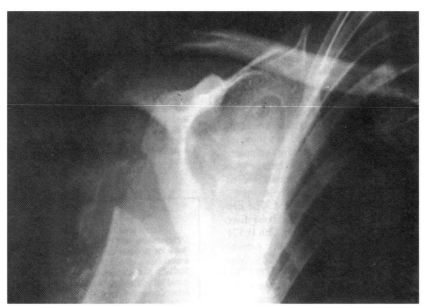

68. A 31-year-old man was admitted to the hospital complaining of increasing pain in his right shoulder. Twelve years prior, he had had a traffic accident, which resulted in a spinal cord transection to the T-8 level. The patient's laboratory work-up at the time of his admission showed elevated temperature and an erythrocyte sedimentation rate of 32. The physical examination showed tenderness and generalized soft-tissue swelling to the right shoulder area. The right axillary lymph nodes were palpable and painful. There was no ability for abduction of the right arm and increased mobility and instability of the joint also were present. The psychiatric examination reported anxiety and depressive neurosis. A roentgenogram of the right shoulder was obtained.

What is your diagnosis?

A. Giant-cell tumor   C. Osteogenic sarcoma   E. Osteolytic metastasis
B. Neuropathic joint   D. Chondrosarcoma

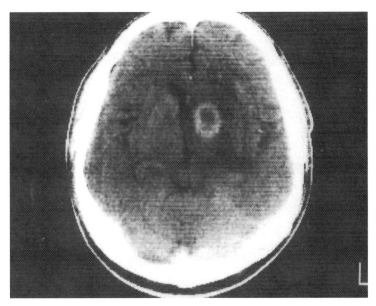

69. A 26-year-old IV drug abuser known to be HIV-positive was admitted with seizures of new onset associated with generalized headache. His CT scan is shown above.

What is your diagnosis?

A. Tuberculoma   C. Secondary metastases   E. Mycobacterium avium intracellular infection
B. Cryptococcal meningitis   D. Toxoplasmosis

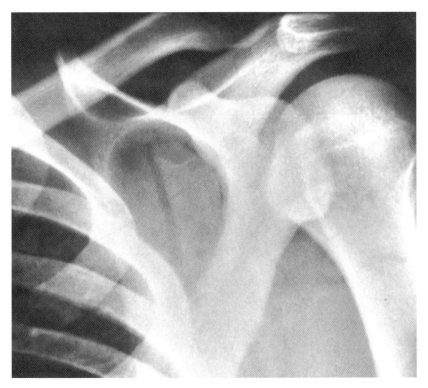

70. A 20-year-old man injured his shoulder in a motor vehicle accident. What is your interpretation of the frontal film of the shoulder?

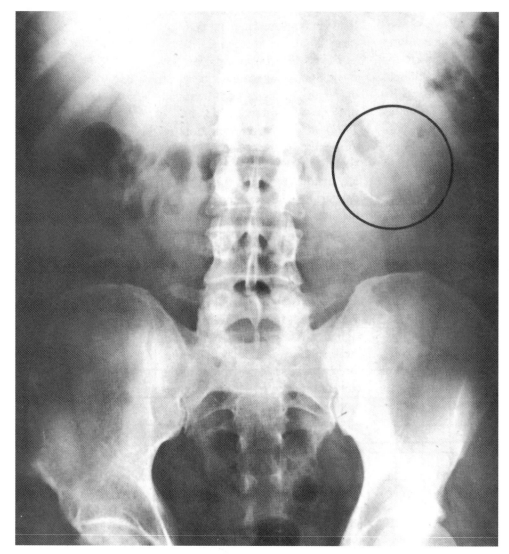

71. The patient is a 47-year-old man who sought medical advice because of intermittent hematuria for one year.

What is your diagnosis?

A. Renal stone   C. Renal carcinoma
B. Renal cyst   D. Renal artery aneurysm

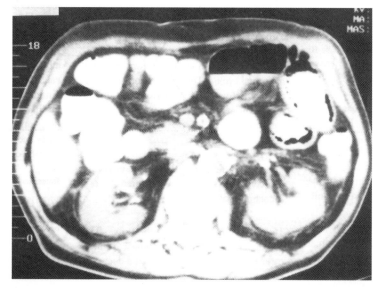

72. The following CT scan of the abdomen was obtained from a 62-year-old man with vague abdominal pain and vomiting of two days' duration.

What is your diagnosis?

A. Normal CT of abdomen
B. Pneumatosis cystoides intestinalis
C. Free air in the peritoneal cavity
D. Gallstone ileus

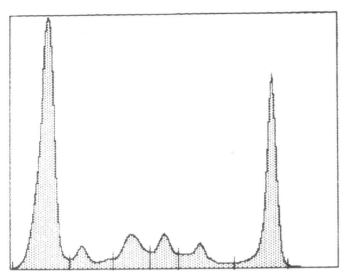

Fraction	Rel%	G/dl
1 Albumin	47.0	3.34
2 Alpha 1	5.4	0.38
3 Alpha 2	8.8	0.62
4 Transferrin	6.6	0.47
5 Complement	6.6	0.47
6 Gamma globulin	25.5	1.81

Total Protein G/dl 7.10

73. This figure is a serum protein electrophoresis (SPEP) from a 68-year-old white male. The pattern is most characteristic of one of the following conditions.

What is your diagnosis?

A. An acute inflammatory process
B. A chronic inflammatory process

C. Multiple myeloma
D. Nephrotic synrome

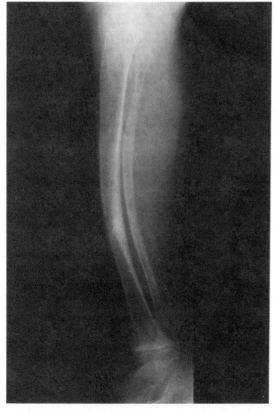
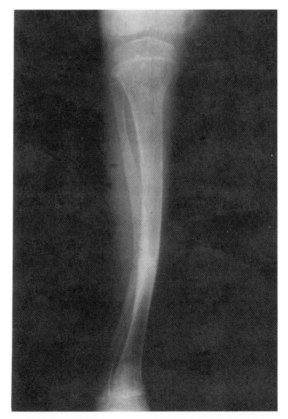

74. A six-year-old girl presented with leg pain and a history of fractures involving multiple sites.

What is your diagnosis?

A. Child abuse
B. Rickets

C. Osteogenesis imperfecta
D. Neurofibromatosis

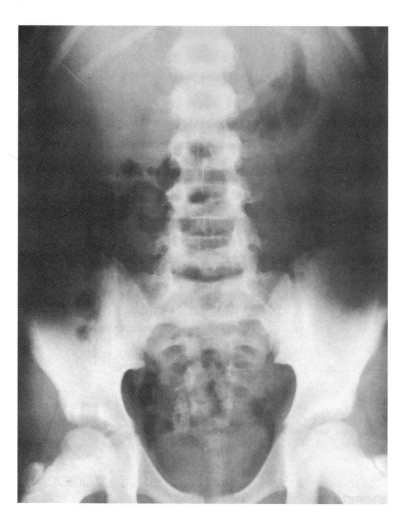

75. A seven-year-old boy was admitted to the hospital with generalized abdominal pain of four hours' duration. His abdomen was soft and his arterial blood pressure was normal. Fever and signs or history of hematuria were not present. Biochemical screening, including investigation for hyperparathyroidism, idiopathic hypercalciuria, hyperoxaluria, and renal tubular acidosis, was negative. Based upon the accompanying kidney-ureter-bladder (KUB) film:

What is your diagnosis?

A. Calcified fecalith in Meckel's diverticulum
B. Stones in diverticula of the bowel
C. Ureterocele with stones
D. Retroperitoneal teratoma
E. Massive calcifying tuberculous lymphadenitis

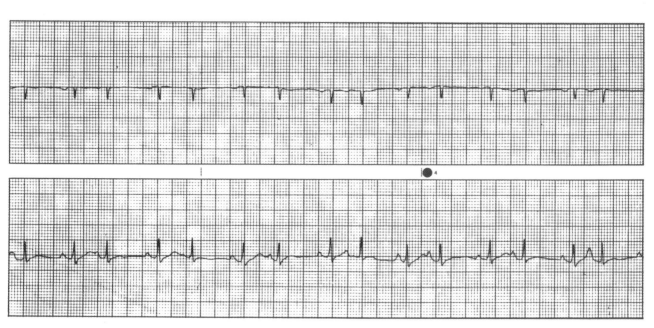

76. A rhythm strip was obtained from a 52-year-old woman following gallbladder surgery. Which of the following is the correct interpretation of this rhythm strip?

A. Atrial fibrillation
B. Atrial tachycardia

C. Atrial bigeminy
D. Atrial arrest

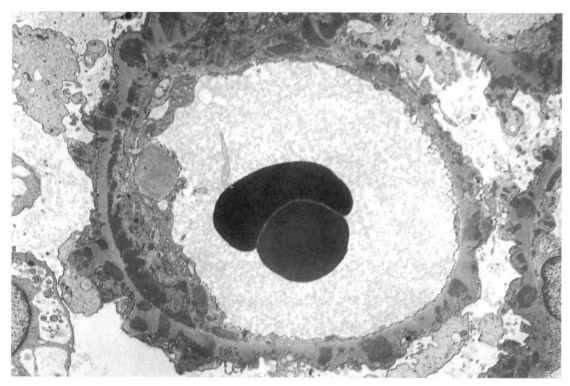

77. This eletron microscopy photograph of a glomerular capillary loop shows features that are most compatible with a diagnosis of:

A. Lipoid nephrosis
B. Focal glomerulosclerosis with hyalinosis
C. Membranous nephropathy

D. Nephritis of systemic lupus erythematosus
E. Postinfectious glomerulonephritis

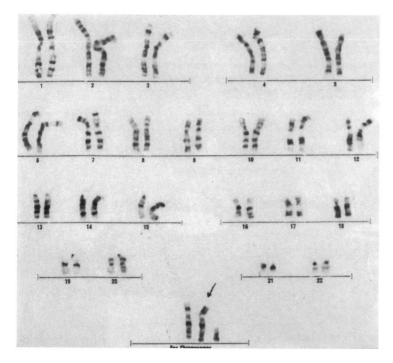

78. A 19-year-old male was seen for learning disability and empty scrotum. His cytogenic report regarding chromosomes from the blood studies is shown.

What is your diagnosis?

A. Turner's syndrome
B. Supermale
C. Superfemale
D. Klinefelter's syndrome
E. Down's syndrome

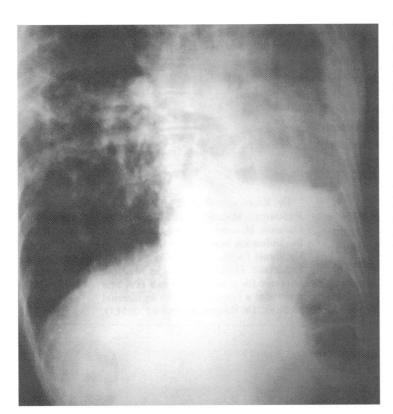

79. A 60-year-old man presented to the emergency department with acute respiratory distress. He was told that he had histoplasmosis. The emergency department physician was puzzled about heart shadow.

What is your diagnosis?

A. Chronic obstructive pulmonary disease
B. Tuberculosis
C. Pneumonia
D. Gastric herniation

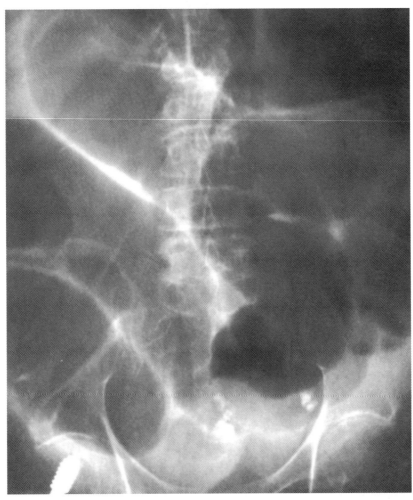

80. An 80-year-old nursing home resident complains of stomach pain. Her abdomen is distended. What is your interpretation of the abdominal scout film?

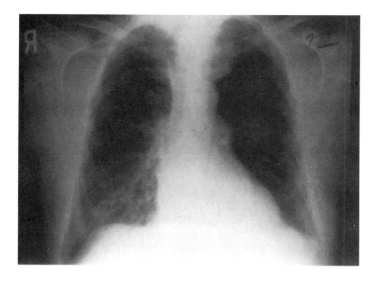
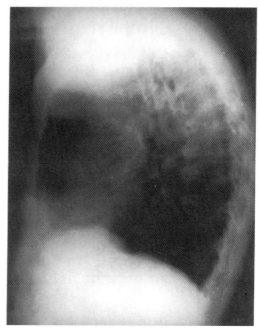

81. A 70-year-old man presented with abdominal pain. Examination revealed a neck mass. There was neither peripheral adenopathy nor myasthenic symptoms. Genitalia examination was normal. Chest X-ray is shown.

What is your diagnosis?

A. Thymoma

B. Mediastinal adenopathy

C. Lymphoma

D. Substernal thyroid and cervical goiter

E. Teratoma

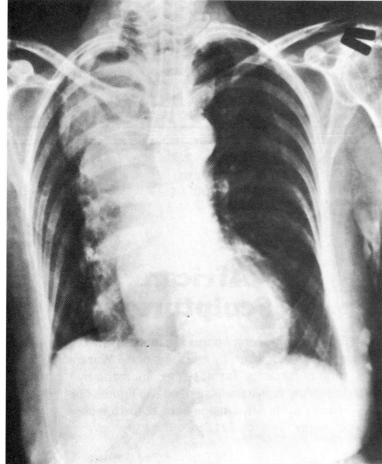

82. The patient is a 67-year-old woman who presented to the emergency department with acute respiratory distress.

What is your diagnosis

A. Lymphoma
B. Achalasia
C. Dermoid
D. Thymoma

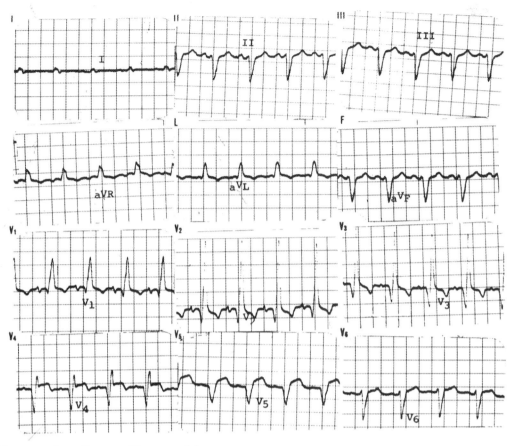

83. This ECG was taken from a 63-year-old man.

What is your diagnosis?

A. Myocardial infarction (MI) alone
B. Right ventricular hypertrophy

C. Biventricular hypertrophy
D. MI, right bundle-branch block, and left anterior hemiblock

Fig. A

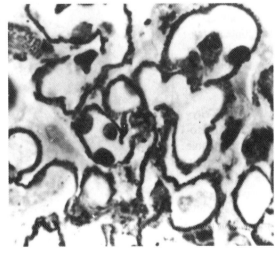

Fig. B

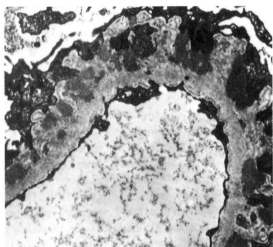

84. These slides are of a 43-year-old man with nephrotic syndrome.

What is your diagnosis?

A. Minimal change
B. Hereditary nephropathy

C. Membranous nephropathy
D. Poststreptococcal glomerulonephritis

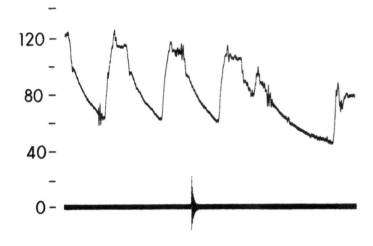

Aorta

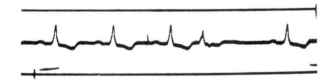

85. An aortic pressure tracing is illustrated on top with an ECG below. Which of the following is indicated by the last beat on the record?

What is your diagnosis?

A. Hypertrophic subaortic stenosis
B. Pulsus alternans
C. Normal aortic pressure after a ventricular premature contraction
D. Stenosis of the aortic valve
E. Pulsus paradoxus

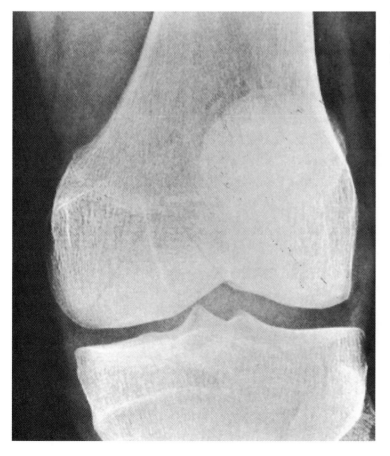

86. A 20-year-old man injured his knee in a fall, and the joint now contains an effusion. What is your interpretation of the frontal view of the knee?

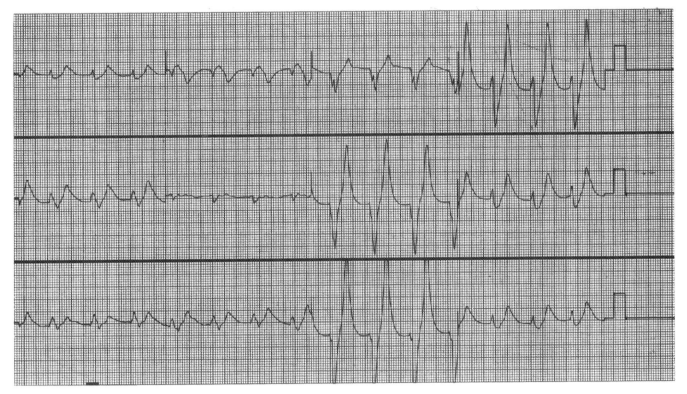

87. This 49-year-old woman with multiple sclerosis presented with nausea and vomiting. Her history did not indicate any significant cardiac, pulmonary, renal, or endocrine disease.

What is your diagnosis?

A. Hypocalcemia
B. Hypothermia

C. Digitalis intoxication
D. Hyperkalemia

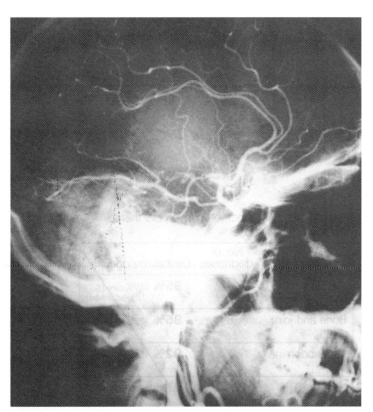

88. A 54-year-old, nonhypertensive man suffered a moderate deficit right hemispheric stroke, with recovery to a residual upper arm weakness. Complete cerebral angiography was performed to delineate possible surgically remediable bifurcation disease.

What is your diagnosis?

A. Ulcerative plaque bifurcation
B. Embolic occlusion of the middle cerebral artery
C. Normal exam
D. Internal carotid occlusion

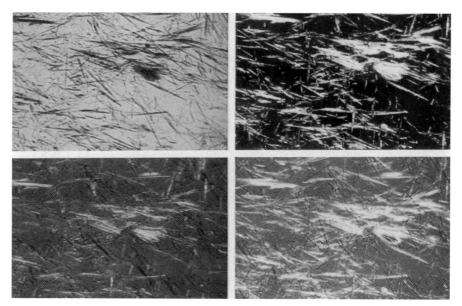

89. A 50-year-old man presented with a swollen, red, and tender toe. The site was aspirated. Microscopic findings of the aspirate are shown above.

What is your diagnosis?

A. Infectious arthritis
B. Pseudogout

C. Acute traumatic arthritis
D. Gout

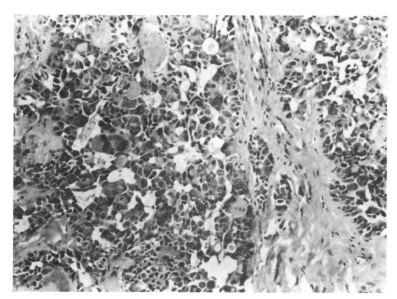

90. A 72-year-old woman was diagnosed as having multiple myeloma. She had been treated with nine courses of chemotherapy and was now stable. The duration of her disease was 10 months. A posterior cervical lymph node, which had been present for two years and recently had been increasing in size, was removed for diagnosis.

What is your diagnosis?

A. Treatment effect of multiple myeloma
B. Paraganglioma
C. Metastatic medullary carcinoma of the thyroid gland
D. Metastatic undifferentiated carcinoma with an undetermined primary site

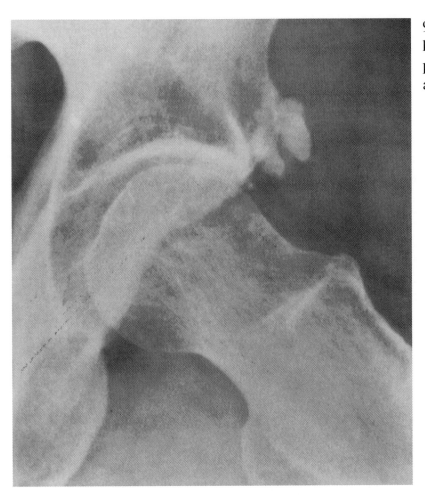

91. A 40-year-old man says his hip has been hurting for the past week. What is your interpretation of this frontal film of the painful area?

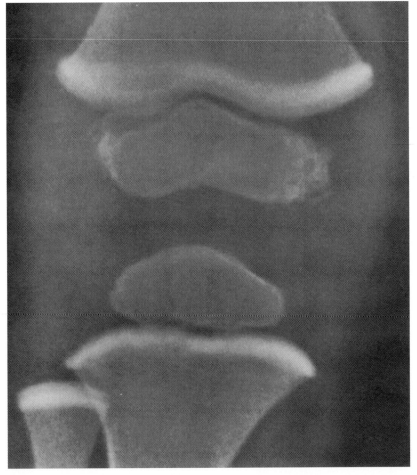

92. A two-year-old child with apparent knee injury is being examined because of suspected abuse. What is your interpretation of the frontal film of his knee?

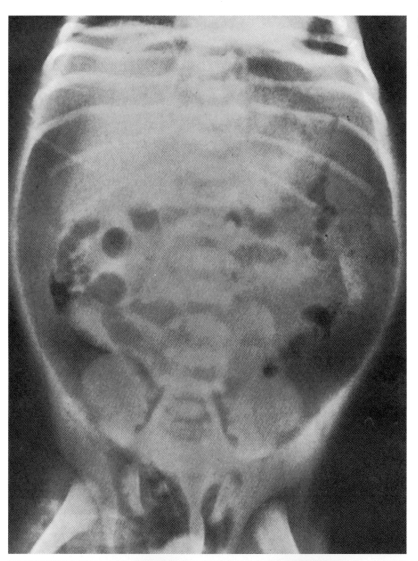

93. The abdomen of a neonate suddenly became distended. What is your interpretation of the scout film of his abdomen?

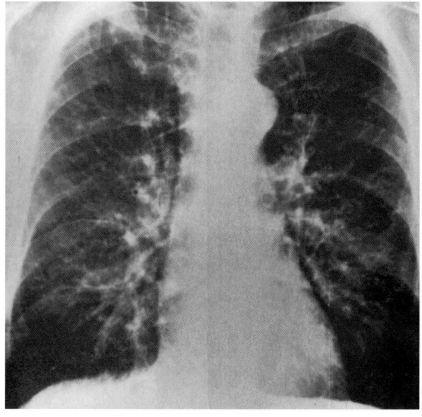

94. A 64-year-old man has severe shortness of breath that has lasted for several hours. What is your interpretation of the frontal chest film?

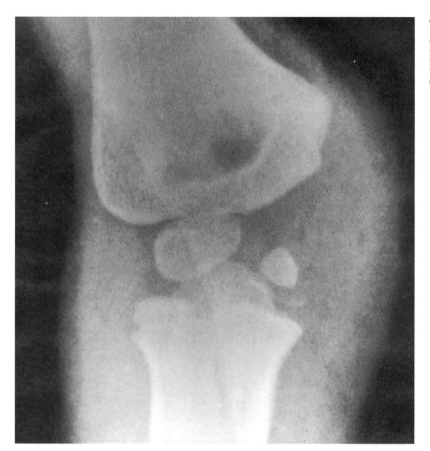

95. A six-year-old girl complains of pain in her elbow after a fall. What is your interpretation of the frontal view of the elbow?

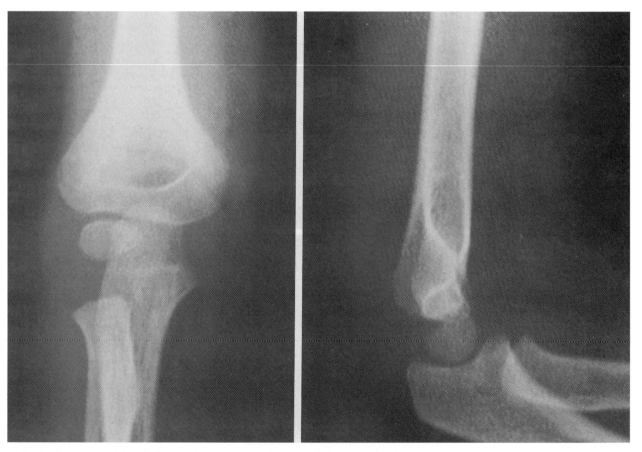

96. A six-year-old child hurt her elbow when she tripped and fell. What is your interpretation of the frontal (left) and lateral (right) films?

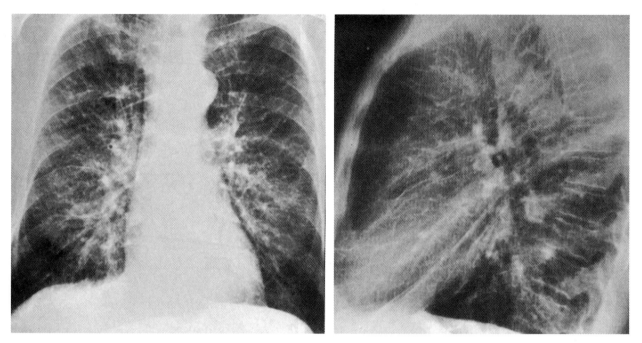

97. A 64-year-old man complains of severe chest pain and shortness of breath of two hours' duration. What is your interpretation of his AP (left) and lateral (right) chest films?

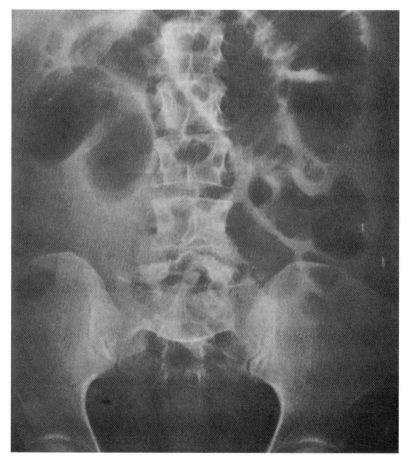

98. A 17-year-old boy has had diffuse abdominal pain for six hours. What is your interpretation of the scout film of his abdomen?

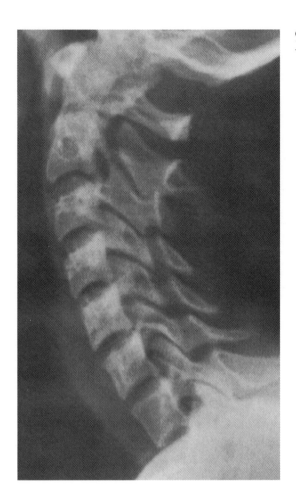

99. A 16-year-old boy injured his neck in a motor vehicle accident. What is your interpretation of the lateral view of his cervical spine?

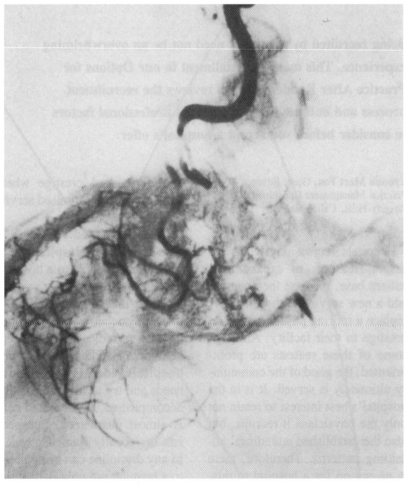

100. A 58-year-old, hypertensive man was evaluated for a bilateral nonspecific decrease in visual acuity. Noninvasive cerebrovascular examination was unremarkable, as was the ophthalmologic examination. Therefore, complete cerebral angiography was obtained.

What is your diagnosis?

A. Internal carotid artery occlusion
B. Vertebral artery occlusion
C. Basilar artery occlusion
D. Ulcerative plaque bifurcation

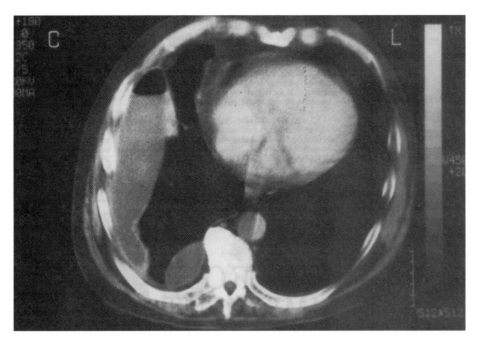

101. A 35-year-old diabetic man presented with fever and chills of ten days' duration. After the initial chest x-ray, a computerized tomography (CT) scan of the chest was taken.

What is your diagnosis?

A. Lung abscess   C. Cavitary bronchogenic carcinoma
B. Empyema   D. Mesothelioma

PHOTO DIAGNOSIS

ANSWERS

Vol. 2

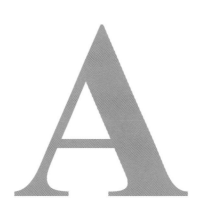

1. **The clinical diagnosis is pyogenic granuloma.** Trauma and secondary infection precipitate formation of the rapidly growing 0.5- to 1.5-cm, sharply demarcated nodules, which are fleshy and pedunculated and may be bright red to violaceous. The slightest injury to the friable lesions results in profuse bleeding. The commonest site is the fingers, but they may develop on other extremities and the face. Children are most often affected. If not completely destroyed, the lesions will invariably recur, and thorough curettage under local anesthesia must be followed by electrodesiccation. Excision by tunable dye laser is also effective.

2. **The correct diagnosis is seminoma.** Typically occurring in an older age group than non-seminomatous tumors, seminomas are also of lower malignant potential. Whereas embryonal carcinoma is derived from primordial germ cells and spermatogia, seminoma originates from spermatocytes, and the differentiation in the tumor recapitulates spermatogenesis. Seminomas consist of sheets of relatively monomorphous, round cells with distinct nucleoli. Lymphoid infiltration of the stroma is common, and occasionally granulomas are present. Giant cells resembling syncytiotrophoblasts and containing human chorionic gonadotropin may be present and may augur a worse prognosis. Seminomas account for about 40% of all testicular neoplasms and are extremely radiosensitive.

3. **The diagnosis is tinea versicolor**, a superficial fungal infection of the stratum corneum. The noninflammatory macular patches range from white to yellowish brown to dark brown. If scaling is not initially seen, it will become apparent when the skin surface is gently scratched. The infection is differentiated from tinea corporis--ringworm of the glabrous skin--by the absence of inflammation and elevated borders. The lesions of vitiligo lack melanocytes and thus are usually white. They are prone to sunburn, sharply demarcated, and often symmetrical. The macular eruption of secondary syphilis may show some pigmentary change, but the lesions are never scaly. Other secondary syphilitic skin lesions may also be seen. To confirm the diagnosis of tinea versicolor, examine a potassium hydroxide preparation of some skin scrapings under a microscope. You will see the characteristic morphology of *Pityrosporum orbiculare*: numerous short, plump mycelia (hyphae) and spores that together resemble spaghetti and meatballs. The fungus on the skin appears as a golden fluorescence under Wood's light, a useful tool for demonstrating the extent of the infection.

4. **The correct diagnosis is *cytomegalovirus infection.*** Cytomegalovirus (CMV) is one of the most common infective agents detected in patients with acquired immunodeficiency syndrome (AIDS). In gastrointestinal tract infections, CMV is the most common causative agent diagnosed by tissue biopsy. The colon and esophagus are frequently affected sites. CMV-related tissue damage is probably due to vasculitis. Odynophagia, dysphagia, and upper gastrointestinal hemorrhages are the common presenting symptoms. Tissue diagnosis is dependent on the typical viral cytopathic changes, that is, enlarged nucleus with intranuclear and cytoplasmic inclusions. The herpetic infection produces a large cell with multiple nuclei showing margination and molding. Immunoperoxidase and in situ hybridization techniques facilitate a definitive diagnosis of CMV infection when tissue changes are equivocal. The availability of ganciclovir (Cytovene®) for successful treatment of CMV infection makes an early diagnosis of the disease by all available means necessary.

5. **The correct diagnosis is Reiter's syndrome.** This HLA-B27-positive patient had a severe case of endemic (genitourinary) Reiter's syndrome, manifested by keratoderma blennorrhagia, circinate balanitis, painless oral lesions, urethritis, and erosive arthritis of the interphalangeal joint of the great toe.

6. **The correct diagnosis is *early thioridazine toxicity*.** Like other phenothiazines, thioridazine selectively accumulates in the uveal melanin, and unlike others, it is toxic to the visual cell enzymes in relatively high concentrations, and thus, may cause retinopathy. Thioridazine retinopathy has a very characteristic clinical picture. Initial complaints of brownish-colored vision, blurred vision, or decreased night vision may precede funduscopic abnormalities by days or weeks. Then the fundi begin to show fine, diffuse "salt and pepper" pigmentary granulation. Gradually, the dark pigment granules coarsen and coalesce into large clumps or plaques, sometimes continuing even after drug discontinuation. Thioridazine should be discontinued promptly after recognition of the clinical symptoms or the funduscopic pigmentation.

7. **The correct diagnosis is *granulosa cell tumor*.** Granulosa cell tumor is the most common clinically estrogenic ovarian tumor, and it occurs more often in postmenopausal women. It is unilateral in 95% of cases. Characteristically, the tumor is predominantly cystic with solid areas, and its size averages 12 cm. The cystic compartments are typically filled with hemorrhagic fluid or clotted blood. Histologically, it consists of granulosa, or more often, granulosa and theca cells. The theca cells are believed to be a reactive proliferation to granulosa cell growth. The granulosa cells may be arranged in various patterns, commonly admixed, such as microfollicular with small cavities filled with eosinophilic material, macrofollicular trabecular, hollow tubular, solid tubular, and diffuse.

8. **The correct diagnosis is *condylomata acuminata*.** Condylomata acuminata are venereal warts caused by the human papilloma virus. The lesions usually begin as soft, flesh-colored, flat or ragged papules. They may coalesce to form velvety plaques, discrete warty papules, or cauliflower-like growths. Condylomata acuminata are often located in the perianal region, around the edges of the labia and introitus, or on the glans or shaft of the penis. Transmission is usually by sexual contact. Occasionally, transmission may be by close family contact or during delivery by passage through an infected birth canal. Occurrence of these lesions in prepubertal children should raise questions regarding the possibility of abuse. The treatment of condylomata acuminata consists of the topical application of podophyllin.

    The lesions of molluscum contagiosum are discrete, waxy, dome-shaped papules with central umbilication. Genital herpes lesions are caused by herpes simplex type II and are found in the genital areas. In genital herpes, the lesions are vesicular. In later stages, shallow, painful lacerations may be found. The lesions of condylomata lata (the Latin word *lata* means "broad" or "flat") of secondary syphilis may be distinguished from the lesions of condylomata acuminata by a flat-topped appearance.

9. **The correct diagnosis is mitral valve prolapse.** The examination revealed a midsystolic click and a late systolic murmur. The echocardiogram displayed classic findings of mitral valve prolapse including thickened mitral leaflets and a very pronounced late systolic prolapse. Palpitations are a common presentation in this syndrome. Holter monitoring revealed multiple ventricular ectopic beats and one triplet. Although ventricular ectopy is common in this syndrome, syncope and sudden death are quite unusual.

10. **The correct diagnosis is Kaposi's sarcoma.** This disease has a predilection for the lower extremities and the coloration is typical. Biopsy shows vascular involvement and is diagnostic. Lesions may last for years or may spread, involving lymphatics of the legs or other organs. Lichen planus can look just like this, is usually very pruritic, but a biopsy shows a typical picture.

11. **The decreased skin turgor is symptomatic of hyponatremic dehydration** resulting from the infant's diarrhea and is caused by loss of fluid from the interstitial space. Fluid will move from interstitial to intercellular spaces in hyponatremic dehydration because of the hypoosmolality of the extracellular fluid. A patient with hypernatremic dehydration will have similar signs but relatively well preserved skin turgor.

12. **The child has geographic tongue**, a benign inflammatory disorder of unknown cause. Typically, the dorsum of the tongue is covered with asymptomatic erythematous patches varying in size from 0.5 to 5 cm, each surrounded by raised and whitish borders. The central areas of erythema, which have lost their filiform papillae, are composed of atrophic mucosa. The lesions heal spontaneously, but similar lesions form simultaneously, resulting in a patchy, migrating distribution. Geographic tongue is commonest in children and young adults, but it may come and go throughout the patient's life.

13. **The diagnosis is indirect inguinal hernia.** The groin mass extending downward into the scrotum is caused by a persistent patent processus vaginalis wide enough to admit a portion of the omentum or a loop of small intestine. An increase in intra-abdominal pressure--as when a child cries or strains--will increase the size of the hernia. On compression, herniated material will go back into the abdomen; the reducibility differentiates it from a noncommunicating hydrocele. A varicocele, while also reducible, feels like a "bag of worms." Herniorrhaphy should be performed before strangulation, intestinal obstruction, or venous infarction of the testicle can occur. Bilateral inguinal hernias in a girl raise the possibility of testicular feminization syndrome.

14. **The diagnosis is eczema, or atopic dermatitis.** Eczema is a chronic dermatosis characterized by pruritus, erythema, vesiculation, papulation, oozing, crusting, scaling, and, occasionally, lichenification. In infancy, the cheeks and the extensor surfaces of the arms and legs are commonly involved. In childhood, the lesions are usually more exudative and have a predilection for the nape of the neck and flexural areas of the extremities. The lichenification observed on the posterior aspect of the right knee of this child is a result of chronic scratching. Topical glucocorticosteroids are helpful in the pharmacologic management of eczema.

15. **The correct diagnosis is pneumonia.** The x-ray shows bilateral lung infiltrates, which are partially confluent. These findings suggest an extensive inflammatory process, caused by either bacteria or viruses, or both. The exact nature of the disease could be determined microbiologically or by histologic examination.

16. **The correct diagnosis is bacterial pneumonia.** The photograph shows an intra-alveolar infiltrate composed of polymorphonuclear leukocytes, which are typical of bacterial pneumonia. Viral pneumonia is marked by mononuclear cell infiltrates predominantly in the alveolar septa. Pneumocystis carinii pneumonitis is marked by acellular foamy intra-alveolar material and typically does not include a leukocytic response. Shock lung is marked by alveolar cell damage and hyaline membrane formation in the alveoli.

17. **The correct diagnosis is mesangial nephropathy (Berger's disease).** On the basis of the light microscopic examination of the renal biopsy, you may exclude the first three diseases, which typically present with marked glomerular hypercellularity due to the proliferation of glomerular cells or infiltrates of inflammatory cells. By exclusion, mesangial nephropathy (Berger's disease) seems to be the most likely diagnosis, especially since this disease often presents with microhematuria and proteinuria.

18. **The correct answer is IgA.** Berger's disease, also known as IgA nephropathy or mesangial nephropathy, is characterized by mild to moderate widening of the mesangial areas. The mesangial areas contain deposits of immunoglobulin A. In addition to IgA, mesangium may contain deposits of IgG and IgM, but no IgE or fibrin. Early components of the activated complement cascade, such as C1q and C4 are not found . However, C3, which is activated through the alternate complement pathway, may be present.

19. **The correct diagnosis is *nodular glomerulosclerosis*.** Nodular glomerulosclerosis, also known as Kimmelstiel-Wilson syndrome, is the pathognomonic morphologic feature of diabetic nephropathy. It is characterized by spherical or ovoid hyaline nodules with periodic acid-Schiff (PAS)-positive material located in the periphery and opposite the hilar pole of the glomerulus. Mucopolysaccharides, as well as lipid-and protein-rich nodules, are found within the mesangial matrix and are often adjacent to or surrounding the normal-appearing glomerular capillary loops. In the advanced stage, the glomerular capillaries are compressed and obliterated by the nodules, and the kidneys become contracted due to ischemia.

Nodular glomerulosclerosis commonly occurs in up to 30% of patients with long-standing diabetes mellitus and chronic renal insufficiency. Other pathologic changes in diabetic nephropathy include diffuse glomerulosclerosis, thickening of the glomerular capillary basement membrane and mesangial matrix, and microangiopathy.

20. **The diagnosis is hidradenitis suppurativa**, a painful, chronic, suppurative disease of the deep apocrine glands found in the axillae and anogenital skin. Although the pathophysiology is still unclear, surface bacteria--usually pyogenic--probably enter the follicular orifices of the apocrine gland and then invade the apocrine duct and secretory tubule. Pus fills the tubule, which then ruptures, extending the infection to adjacent apocrine glands. Obesity and a genetic tendency to acne vulgaris appear to be predisposing traits. Other precipitating factors are irritation from antiperspirants and deodorants, local trauma from tight-fitting clothing, and preexisting disease that increases susceptibility to infection, such as diabetes. Hidradenitis suppurativa does not appear before puberty. Systemic antibiotics--1 to 1.5 gm of erythromycin and 2 gm of a cephalosporin daily--should be given until the tenderness and erythema have abated. The application of hot compresses with Burow's solution, followed by an antibiotic cream such as mupirocin, three or four times a day will also help resolve the infection. During the acute phase, patients should avoid antiperspirants and deodorants and should wear only loose cotton clothing next to their skin. If the patient is obese, a weight reduction program should be established. When conservative medical appoaches fail, surgical procedures should be recommended--particularly for the chronic, recalcitrant form of the disease.

21. **The diagnosis is toxic epidermal necrolysis**, one of the few true dermatologic emergencies. TEN, a relatively rare disorder, is a cutaneous reaction pattern characterized by the sudden onset of diffuse erythema and flaccid bullae. The initial eruption can range from local to widespread erythema, to a morbilliform rash, to scattered target lesions initially suggestive of erythema multiforme. Within 24 to 96 hours, widespread small blisters or flaccid bullae of various sizes will develop. Clinically, the skin resembles a second-degree burn. Lateral traction will produce dermal-epidermal separation--Nikolsky's sign. Many areas then begin to slough, and the remaining integument may have the consistency of wet tissue paper.

Numerous drugs may prompt the apparently idiosyncratic development of TEN--most often sulfonamides, antibiotics, butazones, hydantoins, and barbiturates. When a prodrome occurs, it can include arthralgias, fever, malaise, and pharyngitis. More-specific clues are complaints of cutaneous, conjunctival, or oral mucosal burning or tenderness.

Though the use of high-dose systemic corticosteroids is controversial, it is warranted in most cases. Antibiotics are useful only when secondary infection can be demonstrated.

22. **The diagnosis is carcinoma of the tonsil**, the commonest malignancy in the oropharynx; histologically, 90% of tonsillar tumors are squamous cell carcinomas, as is this one. Although the tumor is easily visible early on, the problem is usually not diagnosed until the late stages: Early tumors are asymptomatic until they are quite large, and 50 to 75% of patients have a metastatic neck mass at presentation. The initial absence of symptoms and the nonthreatening character of the late manifestations hinder early detection. In a study by Guggenheimer and coworkers, the mean interval between the time patients first noticed symptoms and their first visit to a health practitioner was 17 weeks. Common presenting symptoms are sore throat, referred otalgia, foreign body sensation, and a lump in the neck. Bleeding, trismus and dysphagia occur in advanced disease. The possibility of underlying malignancy should always be considered in cases of unilateral tonsillar enlargement or lesion, or significant tonsillar asymmetry. The differential diagnosis includes lymphoma, metastases from a distant primary cancer, and AIDS-related Kaposi's sarcoma.

23. **The diagnosis is impetigo contagiosa.** Annular, erythematous lesions with honey-colored crusts are typical of the disorder. Culture of the lesions may produce pure colonies of *Staphylococcus aureus*, Group A beta-hemolytic streptococci, or a combination of both. Impetigo on the face, as in this case, is more likely to be streptococcal in origin. Early diagnosis and treatment are important because impetigo is highly contagious. Complications of streptococcal infection include scarlet fever, urticaria, and erythema multiforme. Some types of streptococci are also responsible for nephritis, which can develop about three weeks after the onset of impetigo. Early treatment of impetigo with systemic antibiotics, however, doesn't seem to affect the development of nephritis. Untreated, impetigo will clear within 10 to 45 days. Treatment includes systemic administration of penicillin or erythromycin, washing with an antibacterial soap, and application of an antibiotic ointment three times a day.

24. **The diagnosis is cutaneous larva migrans**, which is caused by the larvae of nematode parasites for which the human is an abnormal host. Because the organisms are unable to complete their life cycles in the human host, they wander and burrow into the skin until they die. Human hook-worms are occasionally responsible for the lesion. Infective larvae penetrate human skin

directly, and within a few hours a nonspecific pruritic dermatitis begins at the site; within two to four days threadlike burrows become apparent. Sea-bathers, gardeners, farmers, and children are most susceptible to the condition. Oral thiabendazole, 50 mg/kg given as a single dose or twice daily for two to four days, is the accepted therapy.

25. **The diagnosis is ichthyosis vulgaris**--"fish-scale" skin--a hereditary and acquired disorder manifested by a fish-scale-like condition. Ichthyosis vulgaris and X-linked icythyosis account for 95% of all ichthyosis cases. Ichthyosis vulgaris is autosomal dominant, tends to spare the flexures, generally appears after the first three months of life, and is relatively mild. X-linked ichthyosis, on the other hand, may severely affect the popliteal fossae, appears within the first three months of life, is restricted to men, and tends to be severe.

A new topical ammonium lactate preparation (*Lac-Hydrin*) is extremely effective in moderate to moderately severe ichthyosis. The preparation functions as a humectant, increasing hydration of the stratum corneum epidermidis and reducing the hyperkeratotic condition associated with severe xerosis and ichthyosis.

26. **The diagnosis is herpes zoster ophthalmicus**, a disease caused by activation of the latent varicella-zoster virus in the gasserian ganglion. Although herpes zoster may occur at any time of life, it is commonest after the age of 50 and in patients with immune deficiencies. Prodromal symptoms typically include headache, malaise, cutaneous hyperesthesia, and fever, followed in a few days by a vesicular skin rash along the innervated dermatome. Ophthalmic findings are quite variable. Initially, the lids may be covered with watery vesicles and swollen shut, with ptosis and scarring occurring later. A nonpurulent conjuctivitis is also common. An especially important finding is vesicles on the tip of the nose, or Hutchinson's sign. When present, it signals involvement of the nasociliary branch of the trigeminal nerve, which supplies the cornea, iris, and other intraocular structures.

Herpes zoster is a clinical diagnosis that depends mainly on index of suspicion. When ocular involvement in noted, patients should be referred to an ophthalmologist. Although the prognosis for herpes zoster ophthalmicus is generally good, serious complications can occur, such as corneal ulceration, iritis, secondary glaucoma, and cataract. Other potential problems include scleritis, Horner's syndrome, extraocular muscle palsies, retinitis, and optic neuritis. Treating ocular complications may entail the use of topical antibiotics, systemic acyclovir, and topical and systemic steroids.

27. **The diagnosis is perlèche, or angular cheilitis, an acute or chronic inflammation of the skin and contiguous labial mucous membranes at the angles of the mouth.** It is characterized by erythema, maceration, and fissuring of the oral commissures. A symptom of any of a host of underlying and predisposing factors, perlèche may have an infectious cause--usually *Staphylococcus aureus* or *Candida Albicans*--or it may be due to ill-fitting dentures, age-related changes in the oral architecture, licking, drooling, gum chewing, and various nutritional deficiencies, in any combination. Perlèche caused by ariboflavinosis or iron deficiency is rare. A culture taken from the corner of the patient's mouth revealed candidal infection. The eruption cleared in two weeks with the application of a clotrimazole cream three times a day.

28. **The diagnosis is tinea cruris, also known as "jock itch" and eczema marginatum.** This

common ringworm infection of the groin is characterized by bilateral scaly, circinate lesions in the inguinocrural folds and adjacent perineal and perianal areas. The tan or erythematous patches have slightly elevated, sharply marginated, serpiginous, and occasionally vesicular borders, sometimes with clearing in the center. The chafting, irritation, and occlusive effects of excessive sweating and high environmental temperatures, binding jockey shorts, athletic supporters, and tight, wet bathing trunks tend to encourage the growth of the superficial fungi that cause tinea cruris: *Epidermophyton floccosum* and *Trichophyton rubrum*. Mycologic examination of a portion of the diseased tissue will establish the diagnosis, differentiating it from similar eruptions of the groin, such as seborrheic dermatitis, candidiasis, and erythrasma. Treatment depends on the severity of the disease: In uncomplicated cases, an antifungal cream, such as sulconazole nitrate, will usually prove effective after a week or two. In unresponsive or chronic cases, a course of oral griseofulvin--after mycologic confirmation of the diagnosis--should be added to the regimen. Instruct your patients to decrease the relative humidity in the groin by avoiding athletic supporters, jockey shorts, and tight, wet bathing trunks. They should also avoid strong soaps and should dry affected areas thoroughly after bathing. When dressing, they should always put on socks before underwear to prevent the spread of fungi from the feet to the groin.

29. **The diagnosis is rhinophyma**, an irregular, thickened hypertrophy of the skin of the nose consisting of immensely overgrown sebaceous glands with patulous follicles. In the early stages, the skin of the nose becomes red and somewhat hypertrophic. Over a few years, the tip and alae become globular, shallow pustules may appear from time to time, and nodules occasionally form to produce, in some people, a rather grotesque disfigurement. Rhinophyma occurs almost exclusively in men over 40 and is usually associated with rosacea, a relatively common acneiform condition of the face that's often aggravated by spicy foods, excessive alcohol intake, stress, and emotional tension. Surgical removal of the excess tissue is the treatment of choice.

30. **The diagnosis is erysipeloid**, an acute infection caused by *Erysipelothrix rhusiopathiae*, a Gram-positive, nonsporing bacillus that is the causative organism of swine erysipelas. Inoculation occurs when someone is pricked or scratched with the bones of fish, poultry, or animals or the chitinous exoskeleton of shellfish. The infection is common in those who handle animal carcasses in their occupations, such as cooks, butchers, fishmongers, veterinary surgeons, and homemakers. About three days after inoculation, erythema and a nonsuppurative cellulitis develop, often extending irregularly and centrifugally with sharp, arciform, and scalloped borders. Regional lymphadenopathy and hemorrhagic vesicles may supervene. Penicillin is the treatment of choice. Most lesions develop over the hands and fingers, so the best way to prevent the disorder is to wear gloves when preparing fish or meat.

31. **The diagnosis is chronic discoid lupus erythematosus.** The sharply circumscribed, chronic inflamed patch of indurated, erythematous, heaped-up, scaly borders surrounding an atrophic, scarred central area is characteristic of this easily recognized and diagnosed dermatologic condition. The initial papule or wheal is followed by a plaque topped by a fine white or greasy scale. The center of the plaque then atrophies, while the edges progress to form a raised, erythematous, and slightly scaly border. Telangiectasis, central scarring and atrophy, and pigmentary changes may occur later. DLE is usually confined to the head and neck. Though inherently benign, this form of lupus can evolve into the more insidious systemic lupus erythematosus. The cause of

lupus erythematosus remains unknown, but it may stem from a combination of genetic, infectious, and immunologic factors. A drug-induced form of lupus erythematosus is not uncommon, and environment may play a role--half of all patients have been exposed to the sun before onset of the rash. Treatment for this dermatosis consists of either injection of triamcinolone acetonide directly into the borders of the lesion or application of a potent topical fluorinated corticosteroid preparation rubbed into the entire lesion twice a day. The patient should use a sunscreen that provides maximal protection--a sun protective factor of 15 or higher--before being exposed to the sun or other sources of ultraviolet radiation.

32. **The diagnosis is basal cell carcinoma**, the most frequent malignant skin tumor in whites but rare in dark-skinned people. The incidence of basal cell carcinoma increases greatly with exposure to the sun and ionizing radiation. More than 75% of its victims are over the age of 40. The tumors are commonly found on the eyelids, the inner canthus, and the retroauricular areas, although no area of the body surface--except, possibly, the palms, the soles, and the vermilions of the lips--is unsusceptible. They may occur in burn and vaccination scars. The initial nodule--which is small, discrete, and waxy looking, surrounded by a pearly border--may ulcerate in time. The lesion is sometimes pigmented or cystic, commonly with telangiectases--reflecting epidermal atrophy--across the surface. Basal cell carcinoma is the least aggressive of all cancers of the skin--it grows very slowly and almost never metastasizes. A "friendly" malignancy, it's completely curable if treated--usually by excision--before it has grown extensively. Left untreated, it invades and destroys adjacent and deeper tissues, hence the epithet "rodent ulcer."

33. **The diagnosis is erythema nodosum**, which is characterized by an acute onset of tender pretibial nodules on both legs and fever in a person with evidence of systemic illness. The skin lesions may be preceded by an upper respiratory tract infection, and joint pains are common. Diseases known to precipitate erythema nodosum include recent streptococcal infection, tuberculosis, sarcoidosis, and a variety of fungal and viral infections. Exposure to certain drugs--notably oral contraceptives and sulfathiazole--may also trigger the lesions. The disease is three times commoner in women than in men. Bed rest and aspirin often provide relief. Left untreated, erythema nodosum will generally resolve in three to six weeks, during which time new lesions usually appear, especially if the patient remains ambulatory. Individual lesions undergo characteristic changes as they develop and then disappear. When first noted, the nodules are red and slightly elevated, with diffuse margins. They are extremely tender, which helps distinguish them from ordinary bruises. The lesions change from red to violaceous as they develop, becoming less tender as they begin to fade. Because of hemorrhage in the subcutaneous tissue, they have the characteristic color changes of a bruise as they disappear.

34. **The diagnosis is herpes zoster**, or shingles. Caused by a virus similar or identical to that of chickenpox, herpes zoster may affect various cranial and spinal cord nerves, particularly the dorsal root ganglia. Because the affected nerve or nerves are almost invariably unilateral, the pain and itching that result characteristically affect only one side. Although zoster is generally self-limiting--this patient's symptoms lasted for two weeks and slowly abated--the itching and pain should be managed with oral antihistamines and analgesics. There is no known cure, but many dermatologists prescribe large doses of acyclovir--eight 200-mg capsules a day--in an attempt to shorten the course of the disease and reduce the duration and severity of complications.

Postherpetic neuralgia is the most feared complication. It usually occurs in people over the age of 50 and sometimes lasts for months or years.

35. **The diagnosis is oral hairy leukoplakia**, a diagnostic hallmark of AIDS. Oral hairy leukoplakia resembles thrush and is characterized by slightly raised, poorly demarcated, corrugated, fuzzy whitish plaques on the lateral borders of the tongue and buccal mucosa. It's asymptomatic and appears to be caused by an infection with viral (Epstein-Barr and human papilloma) and fungal (candida) organisms alone or in any combination. Oral hairy leukoplakia is seen almost exclusively in HIV--immunosuppressed homosexual men. Since the lesions are asymptomatic, no treatment is necessary.

36. **The diagnosis is *cytomegalovirus infection*--**Cytomegalovirus is commonly found in HIV-infected mothers and their offspring. Numerous organs are involved in immunodeficient patients. Commonly, the cells of the renal tubules contain eosinophilic intranuclear (Cowdry type A) inclusions, which consist of clusters of cytomegalovirus particles. The virus-containing epithelial cells can be demonstrated in the urinary sediment. The infection is usually transmitted from the mother across the placenta. Ganciclovir (Cytovene®) and foscarnet (Foscavir®) are highly active against the virus, but resistance may develop.

37. **The diagnosis is steroid-induced acne--**The rash is monomorphous, affects the chest and upper arms, and often spares the face. There are no associated comedones. Acne vulgaris most often affects the face, has associated comedones, and has lesions in various stages. Miliaria can produce an identical rash, but is associated with an uncomfortable prickly sensation of the skin. Folliculitis affects the hair follicle, usually in areas of increased body heat and sweating, such as the buttocks and trunk, or on the face, but is more localized in presentation. Disseminated herpes zoster is usually seen in individuals who are very immunosuppressed, is more generalized, and will eventually show crusting of lesions.

38. **The diagnosis is sigmoid volvulus**, a disease most often seen in the elderly and in psychiatrically disturbed, mentally retarded, or institutionalized persons. The two enormous loops of gas-filled bowel in the left and mid abdomen represent the two limbs of the twisted sigmoid colon. Note the absence of gas both in the rectum and sigmoid colon.

In sigmoid volvulus, the inverted V-shaped loop formed by the limbs of the intestine is typically massively dilated and devoid of haustra. An ahaustral margin of the dilated colon will overlie the border of the shadow and the descending colon. The top of a sigmoid volvulus usually lies very high in the abdomen. Inferiorly, you may occasionally see the actual twisted loop obstructed by gas--the so-called bird beak sign.

39. **The diagnosis is diffuse gastric carcinoma infiltrating the colon.** Diffuse gastric carcinoma is characterized by its infiltrative nature. The fibrous tissue developing at the site of the tumor results in a rigid, thickened gastric wall. This type of gastric cancer gives the radiologic picture of linitis plastica. Metastatic carcinoma in the colon are unusual, accounting for less than 1% of colonic cancers. They may arise from neighboring pelvic organs (cervix, uterus, or ovaries) or from distant primaries (breast, lung, or skin melanomas), and occasionally from the pancreas, kidney, or stomach. The majority of metastatic lesions from the stomach involve the transverse colon

by way of the gastrocolic ligament. Also, colon involvement from primary carcinoma of the stomach may occur through the lymphatics of the transverse mesocolon. When the colon involvement is far advanced, it often is impossible to distinguish whether the primary lesion was serosal or submucosal.

The barium enema examination demonstrated two involved areas. One area was located in the ascending colon, where the mucosal pattern was altered markedly with a narrowing of the lumen. The second lesion was located in the distal part of the transverse colon. The cranial mucosal pattern was destroyed and concave due to displacement and infiltration, but the opposite colonic haustrations were intact. The cecum peristalsis was increased. There was no difficulty in introducing the barium mixture into the colon, and complete evacuation of the mixture was easy. The diagnosis of this patient was established by gastroscopy and biopsy.

40. The diagnosis is spontaneous pneumomediastinum.

The presence of gas in the mediastinum and soft tissues of the neck is diagnostic. Note the gas paralleling the left side of the heart shadow in the frontal projection (Figure A) and under the thymus in the lateral projection(Figure B). The mechanism of gas leakage in this patient is related to forceful straining with closed glottis and eventual rupture of the lung, with air passing into the mediastinum and dissection of the air into the soft tissues of the neck.

41. The correct diagnosis is heart failure with venous hypertension and resulting cephalization of pulmonary blood flow--diversion of blood to the upper lobes.

The cephalization of blood flow is reflected by the huge veins and arteries of the upper lobes, especially in the right lung. The plump right hilum is another result of the engorgement of the veins of the upper lobe. Cephalization of blood flow is a useful sign of venous hypertension and is most commonly the result of heart failure.

42. The correct diagnosis is lead poisoning. The key finding is the very dense bands seen adjacent to the growth plates. The same phenomenon can also be seen in bismuth and phosphorus poisoning but lead is far the commonest etiology. Children may acqire lead poisoning by eating old window-glazing putty.

43. The correct diagnosis is Paget's disease.

This case nicely demonstrates the biphasic nature of this disease. The navicular and calcaneus show coarsened trabeculation of the bone and enlargement in size, representing the blastic stage. In the tibia, the process is in the lytic phase and shows the typical blade-of-grass appearance of its junction with normal bone.

44. The correct diagnosis is dislocation of the lunate. In the frontal projection, the entire lunate can be seen, dislocated from its normal relationship to the other carpal bones. In the lateral projection, the lunate appears anterior to its normal position, with the capitate behind it.

45. The correct diagnosis is sickle cell anemia.

Several of the x-ray findings suggest the disease, including hepatomegaly, a large gallstone, aseptic necrosis of the right femoral head, and osteosclerosis. The last two are manifestations of bone infarction resulting from obstruction of small blood vessels by sickle cells. Hepatomegaly and biliary calculi reflect rapid hemolysis of red blood cells.

46. **The correct diagnosis is ruptured spleen**, indicated by the mass effect in the left upper quadrant caused by medial displacement of the gas-containing stomach. On subsequent questioning, the patient admitted that she had been beaten by her boyfriend several times in the previous week. The diagnosis was confirmed at exploratory laparotomy, and 2000ml of blood was drained from the peritoneal cavity.

Other signs of splenic injury may include left-sided pleural effusion, rib fractures, and gradual splenic enlargement. Real-time ultrasonography can permit observation of the organ and demonstrate intra- and para- splenic hematomas but not a capsule tear. CT with contrast is usually considered the most effective means of making the diagnosis with the least delay.

47. **The correct diagnosis is perilunar dislocation of the wrist, with associated fracture of the scaphoid and ulnar styloid.** The perilunar dislocation is visible in the lateral view, where the lunate is still in continuity with the radius. The remainder of the carpus is dislocated dorsally. Scaphoid and styloid fractures are frequently associated with perilunar dislocations.

48. **The correct diagnosis is Freiberg's infarction, aseptic necrosis of the head of the second metatarsal.**

The lesion's appearance on this film is typical in that it shows deformity of the head of the metatarsal, sclerosis of bone, and irregularity of the articular surface. Some patients with Freiberg's infarction have a history of trauma, but many do not, which suggests the lesion may be caused by the stress of weight bearing. The underlying mechanism is ischemic necrosis. Healing leaves a deformity that persists throughout life. Surgical excision may be necessary to relieve symptoms.

49. **The patient's clavicle is dislocated**, as can be seen from the inferior position of the distal end in relation to the acromion. Inferior dislocations such as this are relatively rare. In some cases, the dislocated clavicle may become locked under the coracoid process.

50. **The probable diagnosis is multiple myeloma**, a progressive neoplastic disease most often seen in patients over 40 years of age. The punched-out, circumscribed radiolucencies are typical, and although myelomas are occasionally solitary, lesions are often found simultaneously at several sites that may include the skull, ribs, pelvis, sternum, or long bones. The lesions are also similar to those seen in metastatic carcinoma of the breast, and differentiation by x-ray findings alone may be impossible. Myeloma does not usually occur in the lungs, however, and pulmonary nodules seen on the chest x-ray will indicate metastasis.

51. **The boy has Perthes' disease, an osteochondrosis of the femoral head**. Aseptic necrosis of the capital femoral epiphysis is reflected radiologically by a loss of volume of the epiphysis and an increase in density and fragmentation of the femoral head. This view strikingly demonstrates an early sign of the disease: a lucency just beneath the articular surface of the femoral head, known as the crescent sign, which represents gas in a subarticular fracture. As the epiphysis collapses, the articular cartilage expands, so no loss of cartilage is found in the joint space.

52. **The correct diagnosis is calcified uterine fibroids.** The type of calcification seen in this patient is pathognomonic. Not all of the fibroids are necessarily calcified, however, and the uterus may extend far beyond the visible calcification.

53. The correct diagnosis is intussusception.

The diagnosis is suggested by the large mass-like filling defect seen in the transverse colon. The mass represents the intussusception outlined by gas in the colon distal to it. In children, the intussusception is usually ileocolic. The diagnosis is confirmed, and often treated, by barium enema.

54. The correct diagnosis is pseudogout, or chondrocalcinosis, a term often used to describe the radiologic appearance of calcified joint cartilage. It is now known that calcium pyrophosphate dehydrate crystals are deposited in tendons, ligaments, articular capsules, and synovium as well. Acute pseudogout can occur in one or more joints and can persist for several days. Joint-fluid analysis using polarized light reveals rod or rhomboid crystals, which appear blue. Acute joint attacks can be treated by aspiration of joint-fluid and injection of corticosteroid esters as well as oral administration of indomethacin or other nonsteroidal antiinflammatory drugs.

55. The correct diagnosis is calcification of a left ventricular aneurysm or left ventricular wall. There is a clearly defined rounded area of calcification at the cardiac apex seen anteriorly and inferiorly on the lateral film. Twenty years previously, this patient had a myocardial infarction and, at postmortem, had a calcified ventricular aneurysm.

The calcium is not in the right location for a diagnosis of calcification of the mitral valve. In constrictive pericarditis, the calcification usually is located at the edge of the cardiac silhouette and often is more diffuse. Although left ventricular enlargement is present, there is no definite evidence of congestive heart failure on the roentgenograms.

56. The correct diagnosis is miliary tuberculosis. X-ray showed hilar adenopathy, infiltrate in (R) mid zone, and miliary shadowings that can occur with all of the conditions listed. With the patient's history, miliary tuberculosis is the most likely diagnosis. Miliary tuberculosis commonly affects the young, immunocompromised, malnourished individual by hematogenous spread. The patient may present with fever and night sweats, and the clinical picture may simulate viral, rickettsial infection, typhoid fever, or brucellosis. Complications such as pleurisy, peritonitis, and meningitis occur in two-thirds of the cases. Choroidal tubercles often are seen during an ophthalmological examination. Leukopenia is present with an increase in immature forms. Skin tests may be negative. A prompt and aggressive therapy with major bactericidal, antitubercular drugs has to be undertaken because this disease carries a high morbidity and mortality.

57. The correct diagnosis is constrictive pericarditis. The pressure record is characteristic of constrictive pericarditis with an early diastolic dip and a late diastolic plateau, which is at least 30% of the peak systolic pressure. This pattern also may be seen in right ventricular cardiomyopathies. One would expect to see more pulmonary hypertension in pulmonary embolism or mitral stenosis before right ventricular failure and high end diastolic pressure ensued. A simultaneous right atrial pressure would be needed to diagnose tricuspid stenosis.

58. The correct diagnosis is sinus arrhythmia. There are no flutter waves and no fibrillation waves, which excludes atrial flutter and atrial fibrillation. The P waves are readily discernible, and there is a consistent one-to-one relationship between the P waves and the QRS complex, with no variation in the PR interval and no "dropped beats" ; therefore, Wenckebach block is not present.

We do see a phasic variation in the cardiac rate on respiration. When the patient inspires, the vaso-vagal response is a transient slowing of the cardiac rate, which results in the diagnosis of sinus arrhythmia. It should be noted that sinus arrhythmia is not a true arrhythmia as such, and is not necessarily evidence of pathology.

In effect, sinus arrhythmia is most often seen in healthy, active, relatively young people, as was the case under discussion. Perhaps the term sinus arrhythmia is best clarified by recognizing that it was initially described in the cardiac physiology laboratory at the turn of the century during the observation of the phasic variation in the cardiac rate on respiration in the hearts of turtles. At the time, it was merely a physiological curiosity. In time, the term "sinus arrhythmia" became incorporated into the lexicon of the modern electrocardiographer.

59. **The correct diagnosis is streptococcal pneumonia with abscess formation.** Streptococcal pneumonia was the most common cause of bronchopneumonia before the use of antibiotics. It mostly affects young children and the elderly, and follows upper respiratory infection, measles, or other childhood exanthema. The organism enters by inhalation and aspiration, and settles in the lower lobes. The alveoli and airways fill with organisms, red blood cells, and edema fluid. Cavities may develop after four to five days. Peribronchial consolidation may occur.

Radiographically, there is homogeneous or patchy consolidation in a segmental distribution, with some loss of volume. Abscesses and cavities may develop. Empyema is common.

Diagnosis depends on culture of the organism from sputum, pleural fluid, or blood. Complications may include pleural thickening, bronchiectasis, or, rarely, glomerulonephritis.

60. **The correct diagnosis is Prinzmetal's angina.** This is a relatively uncommon syndrome characterized by anginal chest pain at rest and associated with electrocardiographic evidence of transmural myocardial ischemia, i.e., ST segment elevation. It is seen most commonly in young or middle-aged women who have other vasospastic syndromes such as Raynaud's phenomenon or migraine. Pathophysiologically, these patients have reversible coronary arteries. The diagnosis depends on a characteristic history and electrocardiographic evidence of spasm. Sometimes provocative testing with ergonovine (Ergotrate®) in the cardiac catheterization suite is required to make a diagnosis.

61. **The correct diagnosis is perforation of gastric ulcer.** Through a midline laparotomy, a chronic perforation of a prepyloric gastric ulcer (3-cm diameter) was found. Perforation complicates peptic ulcer about half as often as hemorrhage. A frequent complication of ulcer disease is perforation, which occurs most often in the pyloroduodenal area. Less commonly, a gastric ulcer may perforate. Peptic ulcer may penetrate the muscularis and serosa to form a pocket or abscess, or it may extend into adjacent viscera. Barium is usually present in the patient during gastrointestinal examination. This pocket usually retains barium and remains unchanged long after gastric emptying.

62. **The correct diagnosis is mitral stenosis.** The abnormal features of the chest roentgenograms are left atrial enlargement, pulmonary congestion, and right ventricular enlargement. Left atrial enlargement is evidenced by posterior displacement of the barium-filled esophagus on the lateral film and prominence of the left atrial appendage, elevation of the left main stem bronchus, and a double density of the anterio/posterior film.

Prominence of the pulmonary vessels is seen in the hilar area, and the vessels to the upper lobes are engorged with a relative paucity of vessels in the lung bases. Kerley's B lines are present. These features indicate pulmonary congestion and are most typical of, though not exclusively seen in, mitral stenosis.

Right ventricular enlargement is appreciated by increased encroachment of the heart beneath the sternum on the lateral film. There is no evidence of left ventricular enlargement with preservation of the normal posterior clear space above the diaphragm.

Atrial septal defect causes more central pulmonary engorgement without left atrial enlargement. Left ventricular enlargement would be expected in aortic insufficiency and ventricular septal defect. A cardiomyopathy would not be associated with such marked, isolated left atrial enlargement.

63. **The correct diagnosis is Wolff-Parkinson-White syndrome.** The Lown-Ganong-Levine syndrome is electrocardiographically characterized by a short PR interval as the sole electrocardiographic abnormality, which is quite distinct from the electrocardiogram under discussion. Barlow's syndrome (prolapsed mitral valve) and Tietze's syndrome (costochondritis) have no significantly known association with ventricular pre-excitation. The electrocardiogram under discussion exhibits the classic shortening of the PR interval; prolongation of the QRS complex and delta waves represented by slurring of the upstroke of the QRS complexes are most prominently seen in leads I, aVL, V_2 through V_6.

64. **The correct diagnosis is second-degree heart block (Mobitz type II).** The presence of nonconducted "dropped" P waves excludes first degree heart block. The presence of regular PR intervals excludes complete heart block. Additionally, the absence of progressive lengthening of the PR intervals excludes Mobitz Type I Wenckebach. There are regular PP interval with regular PR intervals, so that there is alteration of conducted beats and dropped beats with no variation in the PR intervals. This clearly represents second-degree A-V block Mobitz Type 2, which responded well to cardiac pacing.

65. **The correct diagnosis is obstruction of superior vena cava with collateral circulation.** The two veins show an injection of contrast material into the superior vena cava. Dye fails to enter the right atrium from the SVC but passes via large hemiazygous veins to the inferior vena cava and, thereby, gains entrance to the right side of the heart.

66. **The correct diagnosis is hyperkalemia.** The tracing shows absence of P waves, abnormally wide QRS complexes with morphology simulating complete left bundle branch block. Tall, narrow, and peaked T waves are seen in the precordial leads. These peaked tent-shaped T waves are the earliest ECG sign of hyperkalemia. As the serum level of potassium increases further, the QRS complex becomes prolonged. The P wave amplitude usually decreases, and the P wave frequently becomes invisible as the potassium level exceeds 8.8 mEq/L. When this ECG was recorded, the patient's potassium level was 9.8 mEq/L. Evidence suggests that there is sinoventricular condition; however, the possibility of AV junctional or ventricular escape rhythm cannot be excluded. Occasionally, severe hyperkalemia can cause left bundle branch block pattern on the ECG. After therapy for hyperkalemia, ECG tracing was reverted to normal QRS complexes with minor T wave change and sinus rhythm.

67. **The agent is digoxin.** The rhythm strip reveals ventricular premature depolarizations occurring in singles, in pairs, and with variable configuration. The absence of profound cardiac slowing renders propanolol intoxication unlikely. The absence of QRS widening makes both quinidine and xylocaine intoxication unlikely. Since the therapeutic dose of the digitalis preparations is 50% of the toxic dose, we must suspect digitalis intoxication in any patient manifesting this degree of ventricular irritability who is taking one of the digitalis preparations. As matters turned out, this elderly man did develop this dysrhythmia after accidently taking an extra dose of digoxin for several days. The abnormality was noted when he reported the expected anorexia, and was resolved within two days after withdrawal of the digoxin.

68. **The correct diagnosis is neuropathic joint.** Many disorders have been considered as etiologic causes of this condition, the most common being tabes dorsalis, syringomyelia, diabetes, and spinal cord or peripheral nerve injury.

The hypertrophic type usually is easily diagnosed from the massive juxta-articular new bone formation, the osteophytes, and the osseous debris, in correlation with the patient's history and clinical presentation. However, the atrophic type may be misdiagnosed as an aggressive infection or bone tumor, either primary or secondary. The latter shows no evidence of bone repair but extensive or complete absorption of the bone. It usually is seen in the upper extremities and is associated commonly with syringomyelia or peripheral nerve injuries. The incidence of the resorptive type in one series is 42%. It has been suggested that the atrophic type reflects the "acute" phase of the disease and the hypertrophic type reflects the "chronic" one.

This 31-year-old man was bedridden for 10 years because of spinal cord transection and had not shown any abnormality in the hip joints or in the spine, but developed a neuropathic joint in his right shoulder. The anteroposterior film of the right shoulder shows gross disorganization of the joint and complete resorption of the humeral head with no evidence of repair. Amorphous mineral deposits in the periarticular soft tissues are evident. There is no juxta-articular osteoporosis.

This case cannot be explained on a mechanical basis. It should be attributed to repeated microinjuries of the right branchial plexus due to the patient's efforts to stand on crutches, although neither clinical findings nor patient's complaints were reported in the past. Roentgenograms of the left shoulder and pelvis did not show any abnormalities. A quantitative computerized tomography (CT) of the lumbar spine was performed, revealing remarkable osteoporosis.

69. **The correct diagnosis is toxoplasmosis.** In an HIV-infected individual, toxoplasmosis can present with mass-like effect, generalized encephalitis, retinitis, or pneumonia. CT scan reveals a ring-enhanced lesion characteristically seen in toxoplasmosis, more so if it is located near the basal ganglia. Diagnosis can be established by tissues biopsy. Therapy includes either a combination of pyrimethamine and trisulfapyrimidines or clindamycin (Cleocin®) for a prolonged period.

70. **The patient's scapula is fractured.** The site of the break, at the thin bone of the central portion of the scapula, is the typical result of strong muscle pull by the origin of the infraspinatus muscle. Unlike most injuries to that area of the scapula, the fracture is isolated; usually the neck, acromion process, coracoid process, coracoid, body, glenoid rim, and spinous process would also be included.

71. **The diagnosis is renal carcinoma.** The abdominal roentgenogram revealed a ring-like calcification that was 7cm in diameter within the left kidney. Carcinoma should be the foremost consideration. Approximately 15% to 20% of renal carcinomas will have calcification. Frequently, this will be on the periphery of the neoplasm, giving rise to a rim or ring of calcification. Renal cyst calcification is extremely rare. The calcific ring is rather large for renal aneurysm and there are no other abdominal vascular calcifications. The selective renal arteriogram shows the lower pole renal mass with irregular vessels indicative of a neoplasm.

72. **The correct diagnosis is pneumatosis cystoides intestinalis.** Pneumatosis cystoides intestinalis, a rare condition first described by Duvernoy in 1738, consists of multiple cysts containing air, occurring in the submucosal or subserosal layer of the large and small intestines. The cyst wall is lined by cuboidal cells. Although the exact etiology of this disease is not known, the following conditions have been associated with pneumatosis cystoides intestinalis: pyloric stenosis, needle catheter jejunostomy, colonoscopy, barium enema, organ transplantation and immunosuppressive condition, chronic obstructive pulmonary disease, and premature birth. There are no clinical symptoms or signs specific to this disease. The course of the disease is often benign and self-limiting. Bowel rest and close observation are recommended in noncomplicated cases. Complications include tension pneumoperitoneum secondary to rupture of subserosal cysts and intussusception of the bowel by submucosal cysts.

73. **The correct diagnosis is multiple myeloma.** This SPEP has the classical M-spike in the gamma globulin region that is found in patients with multiple myeloma. This monoclonal gammopathy is caused by increased production of immunoglobulins from neoplastic plasma cells. Immunofixation electrophoresis showed this monoclonal spike to be of the IgG class of immunoglobulin, which is consistent with more than 50% of the cases of multiple myeloma.

Patients with acute inflammatory processes (i.e.,acute infection, trauma, tissue necrosis, etc.) can have peaks in their respective SPEP patterns, but these are usually found in the alpha 1 and 2 regions. These peaks are due to incresed levels of acute phase reactants, which can be detected by SPEP. These acute phase reactants include alpha-1-antitrypsin, which is in the alpha 1 region, and haptoglobin, which is in the alpha 2 region. There is also a concurrent reduction in serum albumin.

Chronic inflammatory processes (i.e., systemic lupus erythematosus, rheumatoid arthritis, hepatic cirrhosis, etc.) can have increased levels of gamma globulin, but these are polyclonal and produce a broad band in the gamma region. Patients with hepatic cirrhosis can have bridging of the beta (tranferrin+complement) and gamma regions, making the two indistinguishable from each other.

Patients with nephrotic syndrome will have decreased levels of serum albumin due to renal losses. In addition to this, a peak in the alpha-2-region of the SPEP will often be identified. This peak is due to the relative increase in alpha-2-macroglobulin, which is a large molecular weight protein that is not easily filtered through a damaged glomerulus. This increase is magnified by the loss of other lower molecular weight proteins into the urine.

74. **The correct diagnosis is osteogenesis imperfecta.** The important roentgen findings in osteogenesis imperfecta are fractures and osteopenia. The fractures usually heal well, but there are some patients in whom nonunion is seen. The repeated fractures often lead to deformities. This

child had blue sclera, as do most patients with osteogenesis imperfecta. Neurofibromatosis could cause radiographic findings in the tibia, very similar to that shown, but it would be unlikely to produce fractures of multiple bones.

75. **The correct diagnosis is ureterocele with stones.** The simple ureterocele is a congenital cystic dilatation of the lower end of the ureter. It is situated within the bladder at the point of the normal ureteral orifice and is encountered most commonly in adult women. Ureteral duplication is sometimes associated, but this happens more commonly in case of ectopic ureterocele in infancy. The most widely accepted theory that adequately explains the ureterocele is based on the persistence of Chwalle's membrane, which covers the ureteral orifice until two months of age. The replication of the mucosa may cause partial obstruction, resulting in varying degrees of hydroureter and hydronephrosis.

76. **The diagnosis is atrial bigeminy.** Atrial fibrillation is characterized by an irregular rhythm with no readily discernible P waves. Since we can see P waves, atrial fibrillation is not a consideration. Atrial tachycardia is a rapid, regular, supraventricular tachyarrhythmia. Since the strip under consideration is irregular, atrial tachycardia can be ruled out. In atrial arrest, no activity of the atria would be visible, which is not the case in the rhythm strip under discussion. What we do see are sinus beats alternating with atrial premature contractions forming a consistent pattern of atrial bigeminy. This arrhythmia was not present on the preoperative electrocardiogram, and it resolved spontaneously after a few hours of observation.

77. **The diagnosis is nephritis of systemic lupus erythematosus.** The capillary contains several dense immune complex deposits located on the subepithelial side of the basement membrane. Such deposits may be seen in many immune complex-mediated diseases, such as postinfectious glomerulonephritis and membranous nephropathy. These diseases do not show the subendothelial deposits characteristic of the nephritis of systemic lupus erythematosus. Mesangial deposits provide additional support to the diagnosis of lupus nephritis. In lipoid nephrosis, also known as minimal change disease or nil disease, and focal glomerulosclerosis with hyalinosis, there are no such osmiophilic dense deposits in the basement membrane of the glomerular capillary loops.

78. **The diagnosis is Klinefelter's Syndrome.** This chromosomal pattern is typical of Klinefelter's syndrome, with the abnormal sex chromosome consisting of two XX and Y components. The most frequent clinical features of Klinefelter's syndrome is small size of the testes (often not palpable in the scrotal sac), sterility, gyneocomastia, skeletal features that are eunuchoidal, mental retardation, psychopathic behavior, and there is often evidence of poor social adaptation. Urinary gonadotrophics are increased with elevated levels of FSH. Chronic pulmonary disease, varicose veins, and glucose intolerance is increasingly seen in patients with Klinefelter's syndrome. Chromosomal abnormality in the sex chromosome is characterized by XXY sex chromosome constitution. The chromosome number is 47.

79. **Chronic obstructive pulmonary disease (COPD)**--The appearance is one of an end-stage lung disease with disorganization of lung architecture in both right and left lung fields. There is evidence of considerable chronic volume loss on the left with shift of the heart into the left hemithorax. The right lobe is seen considerably expanded in compensation. There is considerable pleural thickening on the left. There appears to be an air fluid level with a large cavity on the left.

80. **The correct diagnosis is sigmoid volvulus.** Distention of the entire colon abruptly terminates in a sharp point (arrow) at the level of the sigmoid. That configuration, the "bird beak" sign, denotes the site of twisted bowel and is pathognomonic of sigmoid volvulus. The disorder is often found in elderly patients with redundant colons, and the diagnosis is easily confirmed by a barium enema.

81. **The diagnosis is substernal thyroid and cervical goiter.** Chest x-ray shows anterior mediastinal mass with compression of trachea. The patient had a long history of goiter. Thyroid functions were normal. Thyroid ultrasound showed multinodular goiter, and thyroid scan did not reveal any uptake. Abdominal pain was due to pancreatitis.

82. **The correct diagnosis is achalasia.** Note the air fluid level in the right apex, which none of the other choices could have. The right heart border is not obscured, and the mass is very lobulated and entirely right-sided. The mass must be posterior, but there is no rib destruction in spite of the size. UGI done later outlines the esophagus, as well as shows a small amount of aspiration, a commonly associated findings. Surprisingly, not infrequently there is little history of dysphagia.

83. **The correct diagnosis is myocardial infarction, right bundle-branch block, and left anterior hemiblock.** The Q waves in V_1-V_4 and the OS in V_5 indicate myocardial infarction. The delayed R wave in a VR, V_1-V_3 and the deep S wave in V_6 indicate right bundle-branch block. The abnormal left axis deviation indicates left anterior hemiblock.

84. **The correct diagnosis is membranous (Epimembranous) nephropathy.** The reticulin stain of renal glomerulus (Fig. A) shows an irregularly thickened capillary basement membrane with characteristic perpendicular projections (spikes). The electron micrograph of a capillary loop (Fig. B) shows subepithelial electron dense deposits separated by protrusions of the basement membrane.

85. **The diagnosis is hypertrophic subaortic stenosis.** In hypertrophic subaortic stenosis, the beat following the pause after a premature ventricular contraction shows a lowered pulse pressure and usually a lowered systolic pressure (Brockenbrough effect). This is clearly shown in the illustration. Normally, or with aortic valve stenosis, the pulse pressure in the beat after a pause is either unchanged or increased over that in the normal beats. This illustration does not show a drop in pressure with every other beat, as in pulsus alternans, or exaggerated variation with respiration, as in pulsus paradoxus.

86. **The patient's patella is dislocated.** Normally, the patella will appear in the midline in a well-positioned frontal view, which will show the tibia and fibula overlapping approximately 50%. In this film, however, the patella can be seen to be laterally dislocated. An osteochondral avulsion fracture, usually on the medial side of the patella, will often accompany such lateral patellar dislocations.

87. **The diagnosis is hyperkalemia.** This patient had developed severe obstructive uropathy due to her multiple sclerosis, with a neurogenic bladder resulting from the autonomic dysfunction of her disease. Her potassium level was 11.5 mEq/L, and her ECG revealed evidence of advanced

potassium intoxication. There are tall peaked T waves, absent P waves, and widened QRS complex with sinoventricular rhythm. The disappearance of the P waves does not indicate cessation of the S-A node activity. Although there appears to be atrial stand-still, the sinus impulses proceed to the A-V junction via specialized "internodal" conducting tracts and are able to control the ventricular rate. The patient was treated immediately with intravenous calcium chloride, resulting in the return of a normal sinus rhythm, a narrowing of the QRS complex, and a decrease in the height of the T wave. Further therapy included sodium bicarbonate infusion, intravenous glucose and insulin, and sodium polystyrene sulfonate enemas.

88. **The correct diagnosis is embolic occulusion of the middle cerebral artery.** The carotid bifurcation is normal; there is filling of the anterior cerebral circulation, but no middle cerebral branches are seen. An incidental patent posterior communicator fills the posterior circulation. The diagnosis is embolus of the middle cerebral artery.

89. **The correct diagnosis is gout.** The aspirate was actually tophaceous material, composed of monosodium urate monohydrate (MSUM) crystals, which would indicate gout. These crystals can be differentiated from calcium pyrophosphate dihydrate (CPPD), which would indicate pseudo-gout, by their negative elongation (birefringence) when viewed with polarized, red-compensated light. (MSUM are yellow when parallel with the long axis of the red compensator; CPPD are blue.)

90. **Metastatic medullary carcinoma of the thyroid gland**--The tumor cells show pleomorphic nuclei and abundant eosinophilic cytoplasm. Other areas of the tumor showed spindling of the neoplastic cells and amyloid in the tumor stroma. Tumor cells and stromal amyloid both stained positively for calcitonin by the indirect immunoperoxidase technique. Electron microscopy of the tumor showed numerous, electron-dense, membrane-bound, neurosecretory granules in the cytoplasm of the tumor cells. They were consistent with calcitonin granules. Additional clinical data obtained on this patient showed that she had a previous partial thyroidectomy for "cancer" 12 years earlier.

Metastatic Medullary Carcinoma is a tumor of parafollicular C cells. These carcinomas comprise about 7% to 10% of thyroid carcinomas. Patients are usually in their 50s to 60s. Cervical node metastases may be the initial presenting finding. In addition, removal of the primary tumor may be followed by local recurrences, distant metastases, or regional lymph node metastases, even after many years. These clinical findings reflect the indolent behavior of this tumor, for which the prognosis is intermediate between the follicular-papillary thyroid lesions and the anaplastic thyroid carcinomas. The association of this lesion with the multiple endocrine neoplasia type II syndrome is well known.

In this location, paragangliomas are common. They also have neurosecretory granules at the ultrastructural level. However, they do not show the nuclear pleomorphism seen here and, furthermore, they are highly vascular. Metastatic undifferentiated carcinomas also would exhibit a high mitotic activity in addition to the marked nuclear pleomorphism. Although, after chemotherapy, the neoplastic cells in multiple myeloma can exhibit the marked pleomorphism seen here, they still retain features of plasma cells at the ultrastructural and light microscopy level.

91. **The patient has calcific tendinitis of both heads of the rectus femoris muscle**, a disorder that is identical to the calcific tendinitis often seen in the shoulder. Crystalline deposition of calcium hydroxyapatite can occur at many sites, with the shoulder, particularly the supraspinatus tendon, being the commonest locale.

92. **The child has lead poisoning**, indicated by the dense transverse metaphyseal bands characteristic of heavy metal poisoning that are apparent on the radiograph. Similar bands are seen in bismuth and phosphorus toxicity. The bands typically occur about the knees and often involve the proximal fibula. Similar radiodense lines may be found in the axial skeleton, where they impart a bone-in-bone appearance to the vertebra. The major sources of lead poisoning today are ingestion of paint or paint dust and inhalation of fumes from burning batteries.

93. **The correct diagnosis is pneumoperitoneum, in this case secondary to gastric perforation.**

       The large amount of free air on the flanks is obvious; it outlines the liver and bowel. The linear density in the right upper quadrant overlying the medial portion of the liver and next to the spine is the falciform ligament , not normally visible but highlighted here by the pneumoperitoneum. Gas from the peritoneal cavity also passed through the open processus vaginalis and enters the scrotum .

94. **The patient has interstitial pulmonary edema**, indicated by signs of pulmonary venous hypertension, such as generalized vascular engorgement, shunting of blood from the bases to the upper lobes, cuffs of edema around the edges of the bronchi on cross-section, fluid in the pulmonary fissures, and Kerley's lines at the bases of the lungs. The blunting of the posterior costophrenic angles by small pleural effusions, which can be seen on the lateral view, also suggests the diagnosis. Radiologic recognition of interstitial pulmonary edema is particularly important because early in the disease--before the fluid moves to the alveoli--rales cannot be detected on physical examination.

95. **The diagnosis is avulsion of the ossification center of the medial epicondyle**; in addition, the apophysis has been entrapped within the joint. Stress on the valgus during the fall forced a temporary medial opening of the elbow joint, allowing the avulsed epicondyle to be drawn into the joint by traction from the attached flexor-pronator muscle group as well as the ulnar collateral ligament. The entrapped epicondyle can easily be mistaken for the normal ossification center of the trochlea. In a child this age, however, the trochlear apophysis is not yet ossified.

96. **The correct diagnosis is transcondylar fracture of the humerus.**

       Anterior and posterior fat pads indicate the presence of a large effusion in the joint and are strongly suggestive of a fracture. Further evidence of a fracture is the alteration in the angle between the anterior cortex of the humerus and the capitellum, which is normally 140 degrees. Looking for change in that relationship is very important for detecting a transcondylar fracture of the humerus because conventional projections are often inadequate. The lucency crossing the distal humerus in the frontal film is a skinfold.

97. **The correct diagnosis is interstitial pulmonary edema**--in this case secondary to acute myocardial infarction.

The evidence supporting the diagnosis includes cephalization of blood flow, the presence of Kerley's A and B lines--best seen in the lateral projection--engorgement of the pulmonary vasculature, sharp definition of the interlobar fissures from fluid, and thickening of the walls of the bronchi by edema, best seen at the upper pole of the right hilum. The constellation of finding indicates the presence of venous hypertension and congestion and excludes the diagnosis with which it is most commonly confused--widespread pneumonia.

98. **The correct diagnosis is acute appendicitis.**

An appendicolith is evident adjacent to the brim of the pelvis. Also note the generalized gaseous distention of the small bowel. Some gas is apparent in the cecum and ascending colon but very little in the right lower quadrant. The small-bowel ileus in combination with the appendicolith is doubly diagnostic of acute appendicitis.

99. **The correct diagnosis is fracture of the neural arch of C2, also known as hangman's fracture.** Traumatic hyperextension has resulted in separation of the pedicles of C2 anterior to the inferior facet. The unstable injury is often associated with subluxation of C2 on C3 and occurs commonly in motor vehicle accidents.

100. **The correct diagnosis is Basilar artery occlusion.** This vertebral injection demonstrates a large posterior cerebral filling the stump of the distal basilar artery via the posterior cerebellar.

101. **The correct diagnosis is empyema.** CT scan of the chest is extremely valuable in diagnosing all three categories of pleural diseases: parenchymal lung lesions with pleural involvement, primary pleural disease, and extrapleural lesions with pleural involvement. While a conventional chest x-ray may not differentiate empyema from peripheral lung abscess, a CT scan will. An empyema is almost always oblong, whereas a lung abscess is round. Air in the empyema indicates either communication with the bronchial tree or infection with gas-producing organisms. Lung compression commonly seen in the empyema is rarely seen in the lung abscess. A cavitary carcinoma usually has a eccentric irregular wall, whereas a lung abscess has a concentric luminal wall.

PHOTO DIAGNOSIS

TEST TAKING STATEGIES

TEST TAKING STRATAGIES

Many candidates score lower points on tests than their knowledge warrants because they lack a sophisticated approach to taking tests. Test-wiseness is the ability to use characteristics of tests to reach the full potential of one's knowledge and aptitude.

There are several considerations for taking a test:

- A strategy for preparation
- Stages in learning and studying
- Tips in taking tests
- Anxiety management so that you can operate at peak performance

PREPARATION

1. Study periods are most efficient if they are intense and no longer than two hours.

2. During these study periods, study in a quiet place, and at the same desk if possible.

3. If you start to daydream or need to take a break, do so away from that desk. The desk will become a stimulus for concentration and work.

4. As you read, constantly ask yourself questions about what you are reading — read actively.

5. Schedule your study periods — generally no more than two periods per day.

6. Cramming is a VERY inefficient use of your time.

7. Engage in regular and consistent study.

8. Use multiple choice questions to determine your strong and weak areas.

9. Use a method of reading and reviewing that promotes high retention and recall of specific information.

10. Alternate your study time between hard reading during one study session, and easy reading during the next. This is to maximize your learning time as well as allow you to maintain your stamina in the long run.

11. Maximum learning tends to occur in the first hour or two and then diminishes with continued studying.

STAGES IN LEARNING & STUDYING FOR A TEST

1. Multiple choice questions are designed to assess a candidate's depth of knowledge.

2. Multiple choice questions measure six outcomes of learning and assess five goals of learning.

3. The six outcomes of learning are knowledge, understanding, analysis, application, synthesis, and evaluation.

4. The five goals of learning are knowledge of terminology or specific facts, knowledge and application of methods and procedures, ability to apply facts and principles in a given situation, and ability to interpret cause and effect relationship.

5. The stages in learning and studying for a test are:

    I.   Procrastination:

         "I've got things to do."
         "I'll do it tomorrow."

    II. Chip Away:

         "I'll just read a few sections."

    III. Overwhelmed:

         "I don't know anything. I don't understand anything."

    IV. Recognition:

         "I've seen this before!"

    V.   Identification:

         "I don't understand a specific part."

    VI. Questioning and Expansion:

         "I have two references and they conflict."
         "Why did you do it that way?"
         "Your answer is wrong!"

TEST TAKING SKILL

1. Your skill in taking a multiple choice test is as important as adequate preparation.

2. Multiple choice tests are best done sequentially, in a very methodical fashion.

3. Read the stem carefully, circling key words such as NOT or ALWAYS.

4. Read each of the distractors in order, crossing off the wrong answers.

5. Check the right answer or guess.

    a. Answers with words such as "all", "never", or "always" are usually incorrect.

    b. Longer answers tend to be correct slightly more than chance.

    c. Look for an answer that is different from the others in content. For example, if four answers are about "more damaging" injuries, the odd answer is more often correct.

    d. Alternatives more specifically described are more often correct.

6. After you have decided, read the stem and answer one last time.

7. If you want to come back to a question to think about it, mark it the first time through the test; otherwise, leave a finished question alone.

8. If you are not sure of an answer, skip that one and come back to it later.

9. Answer all the questions you know first and then go back to work on those you don't know.

10. Give yourself a rest period for a minute or two every hour or so, to maintain your mental efficiency at a high level.

11. Learn how to relax while taking a test.

12. Occasionally, rely on your intuition.

13. Read the question carefully to be sure that you understand what is being asked. Pay attention to key words like "most" or "least."

14. Quickly read each choice for familiarity. (This important step is often not done by test takers.)

15. Go back and consider each choice individually.

16. If a choice is partially correct, tentatively consider it to be incorrect. (This step will help you eliminate choices and increase your odds of choosing the correct answer.)

17. Consider the remaining choices and select the one you think is the answer. At this point, you may want to quickly scan the item to be sure you understand the question and your answer.

TEST TAKING TIPS

There are three types of questions:

- The ones you know.
- The ones you may know if you think about them or you know part of the answer.
- The ones that you leave blank — that you do not know at all.

1. For the ones you know, read the question carefully, answer it and do not go back to it.

2. For the ones you know partly, eliminate the answers that you know are wrong and either mark your best choice and put down a mark to tell yourself to return to the question later.

3. For those you do not know at all, put down an answer according to the clues we will be giving you.

4. Try to reason out the questions.
   a. Decide what the key concepts or keycepts are.
   b. See if the answer you choose fits in with the key point of the question.
   c. Circle all the keycepts in the question, such as: *symptoms, lab tests, whether the question is a negative form.*
   d. You may want to work backward, seeing if the answer fits the question.
   e. check for double negatives.

5. Clues to the wrong answers:
   a. An answer that "does not fit" with the other answers is probably wrong.
   b. A wordy answer that is unclear or does not read well is probably wrong.
   c. An answer with the words "always" or "never" is probably wrong.
   d. An answer that is ungrammatical with the question is probably wrong.

6. Check to be sure you are putting the answer in the correct box for the question. Check to see if the answer sheet numbers go horizontally or vertically before marking your answers.

7. Blunt your pencil before the test to make it easier to fill in the circles. Make no stray marks.

8. If you disagree with a question, write your comment in the test book. It will not affect your score unless they decide to discard the question.

9. Pace yourself.

10. If you have no idea of the answer, try the following:
    a. *Similarities*: If two answers are similar but not the same, one of them is usually correct.
    b. *Opposites*: If two answers are opposites, one of them is usually correct.
    c. *Odd man out*: The answer that does not fit the other answers is probably wrong.
    d. *Wordy*: A wordy answer that does not read well is probably wrong.
    e. *Ungrammatical*: If the grammar does not fit the question, the answer is probably wrong.
    f. *Always/Never*: Answers with the words "always" or "never" are usually wrong.
    g. *X-ray/EKG*: If an x-ray or EKG is in the question and you cannot recognize what is on it, read the question and answers carefully.

ANXIETY MANAGEMENT

1. Peak performance involves learning how to control your thinking and learning how to stay reasonably relaxed.

2. Throughout the test, it is **important** that you talk to yourself in a positive tone. For example, saying, "Good, I got most items correct on this page," at the bottom of each page will help maintain your moral.

3. Do not prompt yourself with negative sentences such as "Don't feel anxious," but rather with "I can feel relaxed now" — a positive sentence.

4. Learn to relax in response to a keyword such as "relax." Learning a relaxation response involves some work on your part, but will be very helpful to you in maintaining an optimum level of autonomic arousal.

   a. Sit in a comfortable chair.
   b. Breath slowly and focus on your breathing for one to two minutes. Breath from your stomach area.
   c. Imagine someone pouring warm oil on the top of your head. As the oil touches each of your muscles, focus on that muscle and say "relax." Let go of all the tension in that muscle. In ten minutes you should be able to relax all the muscle groups in your body.

5. Practicing this relaxation response three or four times will start to key the word "relax" with a significant relaxation response on your part.

6. Practicing relaxation responses and reasonable thinking together will help you maintain a very effective test taking posture.

   a. Make a list of five test taking situations and rank order them from least to most anxiety producing.
   b. Get yourself relaxed and imagine yourself in situation one.
   c. As you become anxious, say "relax" to yourself, and then say "I've worked hard preparing and I'll do the best I can," or some other reasonable statement.
   d. After you have become relaxed, again imagine yourself in the above situation. Repeat this process until imagining this situation only elicits relaxation and coping self statements.
   e. Continue through your hierarchy until you overcome the most anxiety producing situation.

7. If you toughen yourself with these kinds of exercises, you will be much more resistant to anxiety and will not become demoralized while taking a test.

8. Your anxiety level is likely to peak as a test date draws near.

9. Your attitude, both before and during a test, can affect your score.

10. A negative attitude will foster procrastination before a test and will interfere with your performance during a test.

11. A positive attitude will facilitate your preparatory efforts and enhance your performance during a test.

12. Get plenty of sleep.

13. Engage in some form of exercise.

14. Eat more fiber foods and less sugar and fat.

15. Do not study the last day or two before a test.

ON THE DAY OF A TEST

1. Get plenty of sleep on the night prior to a test.

2. Do not study at all that morning.

3. Your ability to answer questions correctly will be greater with a good rest because your analytical ability will be high and not overridden by specific recall which are acquired studying on the morning of a test.

4. Arrive early after eating a good breakfast.

5. When you go to your seat, take a moment to stretch and breath. Say some reasonable supporting statement to yourself.

6. Answer all the questions you know that you know first.

7. Go back later to work on the questions you did not know or were unsure of.

8. Answering questions you are sure of first increases your confidence in answering questions you are unsure of later.

9. At the bottom of every page or every other page, take a moment to tell yourself to relax and recite some supporting thoughts.

10. Be alert to read the questions, as they are not as you would like them to be.

11. Pay attention to the keycepts in the questions.

12. Think through the questions.

13. Be aggressive in your attempt to answer questions.

14. Evaluate your answers.

15. If stuck, go to the next question.

16. Use time wisely.

17. Read directions and questions carefully.

18. Attempt every question.

19. Actively reason through the questions.

20. Use information obtained from other questions and answers.

21. If you cannot answer a question, guess the answer because in the long run your chances of gaining points are greater than your chances of losing points.

22. There is sound research to show that if you learn to take tests skillfully, keep your moral high and keep your anxiety low — you will significantly increase your test score.

23. If you are seriously anxious, seek professional help from someone particularly skilled at anxiety management reduction.

24. Under no circumstances do we recommend that you focus your attention on test-taking techniques at the expense of studying the academics of a test. If your knowledge base is lacking, no amount of test-taking skill is going to result in a passing score. In addition, these techniques do not work all the time.

SUGGESTED READING

EMERGENCY MEDICINE

1. *Current Practice Of Emergency Medicine,* Callaham; B.C. Decker.
2. *Current Emergency Diagnosis & Treatment,* Ho Mary T, Saunders Charles E.; Appleton & Lange.
3. *Emergency Medicine: Concepts And Clinical Practice,* Rosen, Baker, Barkin; Mosby Yearbook.
4. *Principles And Practice Of Emergency Medicine,* Schwatz, Cayten, Mangelsen, Mayer, Hanke; Lea & Febiger.
5. *Emergency Medicine: A Comprehensive Study Guide,* Tintinalli, Krome, Ruiz; McGraw-Hill Book Company.

INTERNAL MEDICINE

1. *Textbook Of Internal Medicine,* Kelly; J.B. Lippincott.
2. *Internal Medicine,* Jay H. Sten; Mosby Yearbook.
3. *Essentials Of Internal Medicine,* Kelly; Lippincott.
4. *The Merck Manual Of Diagnosis And Therapy,* Berknow, Fletcher; Merck, Sharp & Dohme Research Laboratories.
5. *Harrison's Principle Of Internal Medicine,* Wilson, Braunwald; McGraw-Hill, Inc.
6. *Cecil Textbook Of Medicine,* Wyngaarden, Smith, Bennett; WB Saunders Company.

OBSTETRICS & GYNECOLOGY

1. *Novak Textbook Of Gynecology,* Jons, Wentz, Burnett; Williams & Wilkins.
2. *Obstetrics: Normal & Problem Pregnancies,* Cabbe, Niebyl, Simpson; Churchill Livingstone.
3. *Williams Obstetrics,* Cunningham, MacDonald, Grant; Appleton & Lange.
4. *Comprehensive Gynecology,* Droegemueller, Herbst; Mosby Yearbook.
5. *Obstetrics And Gynecology,* Wilson, Carrington; Mosby Yearbook.

PEDIATRICS

1. *Rudolph's Pediatrics,* Rudolph, Hoffman; Appelton & Lange.
2. *Nelson Essentials Of Pediatrics,* Behrman, Cliegman; Saunders.
3. *Primary Pediatric Care,* Hoekelman, Friedman, Nelson, Seidel; Mosby Yearbook.
4. *Pediatric Therapy,* Eichenwald, Ströder; Mosby Yearbook.
5. *Pediatric Emergency Medicine,* Barkin, Asch, Caputo; Concepts and Clinical Practice. Mosby Yearbook.

PSYCHIATRY

1. *Synopsis Of Psychiatry,* Behavioral Sciences/Clinical Psychiatry, Kaplan, Sadock, Grebb; Williams & Wilkins.
2. *Treatment Of Psychiatric Disorders,* Gabbard; American Psychiatric Press, Inc.
3. *Psychiatric Disorders In America,* Robins, Regier; Free Press.
4. *The Medical Basis Of Psychiatry,* Winokur, Clayton; Saunders.
5. *Diagnostic And Statistical Manual Of Mental Disorders,* American Psychiatric Association (APA).

PUBLIC HEALTH & EPIDEMIOLOGY

1. *Public Health & Preventive Medicine*, Maxy, Rosenau, Last; Appelton & Lange.
2. *Epidemiology: An Introductory Text*, Mausner Kramer; Saunders.
3. *Statistical Models In Epidemiology*, Clayton and Hills; Oxford.
4. *Occupational And Environmental Medicine*, McCunney; Little & Brown Co.
5. *Clinical Epidemiology*, Sackett, Haynes, Guyatt & Tugwell; Little & Brown Co.
6. *Principles Of Biostatistics*, Pagano, Cauvereau; Doxbury.

SURGERY

1. *Textbook Of Surgery*, The Biological Basis of Modern Surgical Practice, Sabiston; Saunders.
2. *General Surgery*, Richie, Steel, Dean; Lippincott.
3. *Surgery: A Problem Solving Approach*, Davis, Sheldon; Mosby Yearbook.
4. *Essentials Of General Surgery*, Lawrence; Williams & Wilkins.
5. *Principles Of Surgery*, Schwartz, Shires, Spencer; McGraw-Hill, Inc.

ANATOMY (Gross Anatomy, Histology & Embryology)

1. *Clinical Anatomy For Medical Students*, Snell; Little, Brown & Co.
2. *Clinical Anatomy*, Ellis Harold; Blackwell.
3. *Sobbota Atlas Of Human Anatomy*, Juchen Staubesand.
4. *Human Embryology*, Larsen; Churchill Livingstone.
5. *Histology*, Stevens Lowe; Gower Medical Duplications.
6. *Essentials Of Histology Text Atlas & Review*, Krause Cutts; Little, Brown & Co..
7. *Functional Histology*, Wheaters; Churchill Livingstone.

PHYSIOLOGY

1. *Essentials Of Anatomy And Physiology*, Seeley, Stephens & Tate; Mosby Yearbook.
2. *Human Anatomy & Physiology*, Carrola, Harley, Noback; McGraw-Hill.
3. *Physiology*, Berne, Levy; Mosby Yearbook.
4. *Review Of Medical Physiology*, Ganong; Appelton & Lange.
5. *Molecular Cell Biology*, Lodish, Baltimore, Berk, Zipursky, Matsudaira & Darnell; Scientific American Books.

BIOCHEMISTRY

1. *Biochemistry*, Styer; Freeman.
2. *Principles Of Biochemistry*, Lehninger, Nelson, Cox; Worth.
3. *Biochemistry*, Mathews, Vanholde; Benjamin Cummings.
4. *Harper's Biochemistry*, Murray, Granner, Mayes, Rodwell; Appelton & Lange.

MICROBIOLOGY

1. *Microbiology*, Davis, Dulbecco, Elsen, Ginsberg; Lippincott Company.
2. *Zinsser Microbiology*, Joklik, Willert, Amos; Appelton & Lange.
3. *Sherris Medical Microbiology*, Byan; Appelton & Lange.
4. *Medical Microbiology*, Brooks, Butel, Ornston; Appelton & Lange.

PHARMACOLOGY

1. *Goth's Medical Pharmacology*, Clark, Brater, Johnson; Mosby Yearbook.
2. *Pharmacotherapy*, Dipiro, Talbert, Hayes, Yee, Matzke, Michaelposey; Appelton & Lange.

PATHOLOGY

1. *Pathology*, Rubin Farber; Lippincott.
2. *Comprehensive Cytopathology*, Bibbo; Saunders.
3. *Pathophysiology*, Clinical Concepts Of Disease Process, Price Wilson; Mosby Yearbook.
4. *Pathophysiology*, The Biologic Basis For Disease In Adults & Children, McCance; Huetber.
5. *Pathologic Basis Of Disease*, Robbins; Saunders.

BEHAVIORAL SCIENCES

1. *Human Behavior*, An Introduction For Medical Students, Stoudemire; Lippincott.
2. *The Behavior Sciences In Psychiatry*, NMS; Williams & Wilkins.
3. *Behavior Science*, Barbara, Fadem; Williams & Wilkins.
4. *Behavioral Science For Medical Students*, Sierles; Williams & Wilkins.